D1357446

Published in Great Britain by Hashtag Press 2019

Text © Sara Liyanage 2019
Cover Design © Anne Glenn 2019

A CIP catalogue for this book is available from the British Library.

ISBN 978-1-9993006-9-2

Typeset in Garamond Classic 11.25/14 by Blaze Typesetting

Printed and bound in Great Britain by Clays Ltd, Elcograf S.p.A.

Hashtag PRESS

HASHTAG PRESS BOOKS
Hashtag Press Ltd
Kent, England, United Kingdom
Email: info@hashtagpress.co.uk
Website: www.hashtagpress.co.uk
Twitter: @hashtag_press

Praise for Ticking off Breast Cancer

I love the honesty and practicality of Sara's to-do lists. It inspires you to create your own - here's mine: be mindful, be grateful, be kind.
Sian Williams, journalist, broadcaster and writer

Sara Liyanage's candid account of dealing with cancer is beautifully and sympathetically written and should prove a useful resource for anybody needing an insight into what it's like to have a cancer diagnosis, as well as life beyond.
Jackie Buxton, author of Glass Houses and Tea & Chemo

Sara's book is brilliant. As a fellow list-lover, it would have helped me when I was diagnosed. Friendly, witty and incredibly useful.
Liz O'Riordan, breast surgeon, TED speaker and co-author of The Complete Guide to Breast Cancer: How to Feel Empowered and Take Control

Ticking Off Breast Cancer is a candid, thoughtful account of the way Sara dealt with a breast cancer diagnosis. She is one impressive woman.
Victoria Derbyshire, journalist, broadcaster and writer

For L, A and C.

"When you come out of the storm you won't be the same person who walked in. That's what this storm's all about."
Haruki Murakami

Ticking Off Breast Cancer is proud to support
Breast Cancer Care
&
Breast Cancer Now

Cancer is a bit of a stop you in your tracks, play with your head and turn your life upside down kind of thing. Everyone who goes through cancer has their own story to tell. This is mine.

INTRODUCTION

"It's important that we share our experiences with other people. Your story will heal you and your story will heal somebody else. When you tell your story, you free yourself and give other people permission to acknowledge their own story."
Iyanla Vanzant

This book is for you, the cancer patient, and your friends and family. It's about a period in my life when I was diagnosed with, and subsequently treated for, primary breast cancer (which is breast cancer that spreads no further than the lymph nodes and can be removed and treated to a point where the body shows no evidence of the disease).*

Throughout this book, I talk about my treatment and all the challenges that came with it: my worries and anxieties about being diagnosed with primary breast cancer; the myriad side effects that come with breast cancer treatment; the overwhelming kindness and support I received from friends, family and strangers; and how I dealt with my relationships, my children, my home, my family life and work. I talk about how I'm moving on now that treatment has ended; how I tried to find the positives in what was otherwise a rather traumatic point in my life; and my observations and reflections about life in general.

My story isn't special—I certainly didn't have the hardest experience, nor did I have the easiest. It's just my story but that's the point. Everyone has a different cancer story. Despite our different stories, we cancer patients are bound together by the common threads of physical side effects, emotional challenges, fears, mental struggles, but also hope. So, whatever type of breast cancer you have—or had—and whatever your treatment plan involves, within the pages of this book I hope that you'll find encouragement, advice and a little bit of hand-holding.

Wishing you all the very best, with much love,

Sara x

P.S. Always remember that everyone is different. We have different diagnoses; different treatment plans and we react differently to treatment. So, please don't compare your situation to what you read here.

P.P.S. After you've read this book, you may want to hand it over to a friend or a family member who'll be there by your side as you go through all this. Because, no matter how hard these wonderful people try to understand what we're going through, unless they've been through it themselves, they may not be able to comprehend life with cancer. Maybe they can understand a little more by reading this account. I've included a few checklists just for them.

*Current statistics are that one in eight women will develop breast cancer in their lifetime. And of the twelve and a half percent of the population (Cancer Research UK), most will be diagnosed with primary breast cancer. Some will go on to develop secondary breast cancer (where the cancer has spread to other parts of the body and has become incurable) at a later date, and some will get a secondary diagnosis straight away.

Disclaimer

This is not a medical book and in no way intends to impart medical advice. At the end of each chapter I've provided a checklist of practical tips for getting through some aspects of breast cancer treatment. They're tips based upon my own experience and research, which I carried out for the purpose of my website. They may work for you, but equally they may not work for you. Remember that there are plenty of places where you can seek practical advice in relation to your treatment: your medical team, reputable websites, support groups, cancer charities and organisations and friends who've been through it.

Take a look at the Appendix at the back of this book and visit my website: www.tickingoffbreastcancer.com.

Always ask your medical team if you have any questions, or something doesn't feel right.

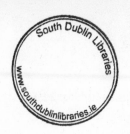

CHAPTER 1

THE SATISFACTION OF A TO-DO LIST

"She is strong."
Proverbs 31:25

It's 7:42 in the morning. I'm in the kitchen on my own. It's blissfully silent. I've made my mug of green tea and I'm sitting at the kitchen table, ready to list what I need to do today.

It's a Saturday towards the end of October and I don't expect my children or husband to disturb me for another hour or so. I'm not writing yet. I'm distracted, looking out at the garden. It has that neglected autumn look about it: damp, muddy grass that's too long; a sprinkling of the first red, brown and orange leaves that have dropped from the trees; fallen apples rotting; and the garden furniture not yet put away for winter in the hope of that last spell of sunshine.

Footballs lie about, alone and unloved. The patio looks forlorn and despondent: yellowing and covered in a combination of leaves, twigs, dirt and garden grime. There's a solitary bird singing somewhere but I can't spot it. It's just starting to get light outside and there's an autumnal dampness hanging in the air. It's the perfect autumn morning to be wrapped up warm and inside, with a hot mug of tea.

4

I have a lot to do today. It's the same every weekend. I don't quite understand how everything piles up over the course of the week and we get to the weekend with a long list of things to work our way through. Surely weekends should be about relaxing, having fun and spending quality family time together? Do other families spend their Saturdays enjoying late brunches, family trips out and afternoons at the cinema? Do they spend their Sundays going for long family walks followed by a hearty Sunday roast around the family table? Or do they, like us, spend weekends battling through homework, driving children all over the place, worrying about the DIY list which is getting longer and longer, doing load after load of washing, constantly tidying and catching up on everything that has not been accomplished despite being on a to-do list for weeks?

I love a to-do list. It's the perfect way in which to regain at least some control over an unmanageable life. Control—oh that wonderful, efficient, organised, sometimes elusive friend of mine.

I love a quiet half hour in the kitchen on a Saturday morning with a steaming cup of tea and only the dawn chorus for company, my husband and two children still asleep upstairs. Solitude and quiet with just me and my list. No demands for breakfast, lost items, or help with last-minute homework. No blaring radio. No loud television.

It's my time to think. Time for my brain to take a breath, relax and recall all those momentarily lost reminders, things to do and things I haven't done. Once they've made their way from the knotted web of my brain synapses, slowly moving to the front like pockets of trapped air rising to the surface of water, they make their way onto the paper: one, two, three, four. . . where each numbered action point can later be crossed off with a quiet sense of accomplishment.

I'm a bit fussy about what I use to write my lists. Today I have a sheet of crisp white paper laid out on the table in front of me. Blank at the moment, inviting me to set out the tasks that will hopefully help me to organise the weekend ahead. As usual, I have a pencil to hand, rather than a pen. I love those pencils with a plastic outer case and thin lead running through, which you twist to get to the right length. But the lead has to be just right. Not blunt. It must be sharp. I have boxes of these pencils hidden away around the house so my stationery-loving daughter cannot find them and I have one of these pencils in each handbag. I would rather leave home without my lipstick than without my pencil.

So, the list for this particular weekend is:

1. Washing.
2. Iron and put clean washing away.
3. Replace light bulb in lounge.
4. Tidy garden.
5. Put garden furniture away.
6. Homework.
7. Unpack spare room boxes.
8. Locate box of Halloween decorations.
9. Order new cushions for sofa.
10. *Get head around cancer diagnosis.*

CHAPTER 2

NUMBER TEN ON THE LIST

"Alone, all alone.
Nobody, but nobody can make it out here alone."
Maya Angelou

Number ten on the list is a new one. Yes, I have cancer and, quite frankly, I don't know how I'm going to get my head around it. Diagnosis day (let's call it D-Day) was ten long days ago.

I would say that up until D-Day, I was a different person to the one now sitting here at the table on this damp autumnal morning. I may look pretty much the same (except that thanks to the immeasurable strain of the past ten days, I'm now about a stone lighter in weight, I have dark circles under my eyes and the startled look of a rabbit caught in the headlights), but I certainly don't feel like the same person.

Before D-Day I could eat, sleep and breathe. I could generally cope with what life threw at me and the weight on my shoulders was that of just an average forty-two-year-old woman. Now, though, I seem to have lost the knack of coping and I feel like a couple of fifty kilo dumb bells are on my shoulders and a heavy chain is draped around my neck.

I was living, up until ten days ago, what one might consider a fairly ordinary life. It was certainly nothing unusual or particularly special. But with just three little words, "You have cancer," the ordinariness of my life seems to have evaporated and not in a good way.

Those three short words have transported me from the wonderful security of normality to an entirely different reality. A reality that I can only describe as 'the dark wilderness of cancer-land,' a place where it seems that loneliness exists alongside fear and sadness. I have left behind happiness, control and safety. They, along with everyone and everything I know, remain safely back in normality and I don't like it one little bit.

Sitting here in this new reality of mine and looking at number ten on my to-do list, I can't help but reflect upon my pre D-Day life. I would say that up until now, I've been lucky, because although my life has been nothing unusual, it has also, on the whole, been a fairly content one. It hasn't been perfect by any means, but since my first grainy Polaroid childhood memories I've mostly been very content.

I grew up with wonderful, loving parents, a slightly annoying at the time but now we love each other sister, and fabulous aunts, uncles, grandparents and cousins. I loved school and my time at university and I now have a lovely husband, two super children, a job I worked hard for, a comfortable home and plenty of brilliant friends.

Whilst it's generally been a very happy life, I now look back and realise it has, especially in recent years, been a rather fast-paced life. One in which I've been blindly rushing along just to reach the next stage: university, law school, a job, marriage,

8

children, a family home and then everything that comes with having a career, raising children and building a family life. I don't think I've really taken the time to stop and press the pause button. Not taken the time to catch my breath or to properly savour one moment before moving on to the next thing. I've always been looking ahead and planning for tomorrow, next week or next year.

With all this planning, every day has become a race. Take my typical day, which I expect is probably the same, or at least very similar to, that of every other working mother up and down the country.

1. Up and out.
2. Take the kids to school.
3. Go to work.
4. Work.
5. Go home.
6. Collect the children from school.
7. Take the children to and from their after- school clubs.
8. Make dinner.
9. Put on washing.
10. Put away washing.
11. Tidy and clean the house.
12. Have dinner.
13. Clear up.
14. Unload the dishwasher.
15. Reload the dishwasher.
16. Get the children to bed.
17. Tidy the house, do the admin, the bills, the organising for whatever project is currently on the go (a birthday,

a holiday, a home project) and get on with all the other jobs that need doing.

18. Go to bed.
19. Wake up.
20. Repeat.

I thought (perhaps conceitedly) that I could do it all. Of course I could juggle motherhood and the work/life balance without any problems, and I was determined to do it perfectly. I was an expert multi-tasker, juggler of many balls and spinner of many plates. Never allowing anything to fall. And although it was busy, chaotic and somewhat crazy, it was my safe can't complain slightly monotonous but mostly content life. Cancer? Well, that has been a bit of a wake-up call.

As I sit here with my cup of tea, I realise that whilst I've travelled through life—running through it at full pelt actually—I've taken a lot of things for granted like my health, family and friends. I've taken my comfortable life, my peace of mind and even my existence here on this planet for granted.

I've arrogantly taken for granted everything that, in the blink of an eye, can disappear. Now, I realise what a fool I've been because, thanks to those three little words, I'm struggling to keep hold of the—what I now know has been a flimsy rather than unrelenting—grasp I thought I had on my life.

I need to stop. I need to press that pause button. I need to take a few deep breaths and I need to think about how to get through this. How am *I* going to get through this? How are *we*—my husband, children and I—going to get through this?

I don't know the answer to those questions yet. Will I ever? But what I do know right now is that I'm on my own out here in this dark wilderness of cancer-land, and I'm terrified. For the first time in my life I feel alone. Scarily alone. And whilst I know for certain that my husband and family will be beside me as much as they can, I'm going to have to navigate this cancer-land all by myself.

But back to this morning. I can hear the familiar rustlings of somebody moving about upstairs: doors opening, the toilet flushing and a tap running. I guess my peace and quiet is over and it's time for the weekend to begin.

CHECKLIST

When Diagnosed With Cancer

It is of course terrifying to be diagnosed with cancer, and there isn't one way to deal with the diagnosis. My main piece of advice for this stage is to surround yourself with your loved ones who can provide the support you need right now. You may wish to, and it is perfectly okay to:

- Crumble to the floor.
- Pick yourself up.
- Take a deep breath.
- Hold someone's hand.
- Cry, scream, shout, rant.
- Take another deep breath.
- Repeat.

CHAPTER 3

HAPPY HALLOWEEN

"She is brave and strong and broken all at once."
Anna Funder

It's now Monday and I'm rather pleased with how much of the to-do list we managed to get through over the course of the weekend, considering my husband and I are still reeling from the arrival of the cancer bombshell.

1. Washing. Ninety percent of the washing came from my daughter.
2. Iron and put clean washing away. Well, I managed a little bit of this.
3. Replace light bulb in lounge—but only after searching high and low for a replacement bulb.
4. Tidy garden. Nope. It rained!
5. Put garden furniture away. Again, not done because it rained.
6. Homework. Let's focus on the fact that all homework has been completed and not that it took cajoling, bribery and a lot of nagging to get there.
7. Unpack spare room boxes. Oh well, never mind.

8. Retrieve box of Halloween decorations. Yes, done.
9. Order new cushions for sofa. Nope, not done.
10. Get head around cancer diagnosis. Still working on this one.

It's half-term and today is Halloween. Halloween is a big deal where we live. Houses are creatively decorated. Pumpkins are carved and lit at the end of a driveway to indicate that trick or treaters are welcome. From six o'clock onwards you can hardly move for the throngs of mini zombies, witches, ghosts and pirates that traipse around with their buckets of treats.

Halloween is my nine-year-old daughter's favourite day of the year. It ranks higher than her birthday and Christmas. I suspect it's because of the enormous number of sweets she scavenges from trick or treating, and being allowed to consume a huge quantity of them the very same night.

I go with the get it all over and done with attitude when it comes to my daughter and her older brother eating their sweets. That way there's less left around the house for them to snack on in the days to come, we don't have arguments about me throwing sweets out, and if they eat a ton and I get them into bed before the sugar rush hits, then we all sleep through it. I doubt I get parent points for this, but it's only once a year and she loves it.

She has her trick or treating route planned already: she knows from experience where the best (i.e. most generous) houses are situated near us. She has her witch costume ready and she's allocated our roles. With my husband due home from work after the trick or treating expedition is expected to have taken place, my mum is going to go out with the children and I'm on duty at home for the hordes of trick or treaters who will knock on the front door.

Yesterday, after locating the box of Halloween decorations, my daughter and I spent a couple of hours outside decorating the front porch of our house with the requisite Halloween-themed decorations: spiderwebs, spiders, zombie bunting, pumpkin lanterns, giant spider lamps and Halloween odds and ends. We carved the pumpkins and lit them up with battery-operated tea lights and we organised an enormous bowl of sugary treats to hand out to the local children who will knock at our door. Despite cancer, Halloween is going to be just as it has been every year.

I'm trying very hard to be brave and strong, to just carry on as normal. We haven't told the children yet that I have cancer and we're trying to prevent them from picking up on the fact that something isn't quite right. I'm trying not to give away that I feel like I'm breaking, that my insides are churning and I can't eat or breathe. I don't want to give away the shaking hands or the feeling that I am having a surreal out of body experience, or the fact that I am scared out of my mind.

So, yesterday I helped to decorate the porch with a fixed smile on my face. The treats were bought with fake excitement and the costumes were prepared with forced interest. Because all the while I was thinking *will this be my last Halloween?*

One might say that Halloween is a good distraction from a cancer diagnosis but, to be honest, nothing is a distraction. Nothing can distract me from what feels like, well, a death sentence. Yes, it really is that scary. I'm still in shock. A time-stopping, mind-blowing, uncomprehending shock. I can't believe it. Twelve days ago, I was diagnosed with cancer. I've had twelve days to get my head around it, but I still haven't.

How did I get here? How did I, a regular forty-two-year-old wife and mother, get to be sitting at my kitchen table with the remnants of lunch yet to be cleared away, on this October afternoon, feeling like I'm about to vomit from fear because I have freaking cancer?

It all began with a teeny, tiny, little lump, which I found in my left armpit whilst on holiday over the summer just gone.

We were in Fuerteventura; the weather was glorious; the kids were playing in the pool and I was relaxing on a sunbed. As I was lying there with not a care in the world, arms above my head, absorbing the wonderful sunshine, I happened to scratch my bare armpit and found a lump. I checked my other armpit, but no, there wasn't a matching one under there. Yes, it was a bit odd, but I wasn't all that concerned because having a lump in my armpit didn't ring any alarm bells with me. In fact, I forgot about it until around a month later. I don't know what reminded me, but as I was going about a normal morning of running errands I checked under there and, nope, no lump. What I didn't realise at that moment was that I'd checked my armpit with my arm in a different position to when I'd been lying on the sunbed. My arm wasn't above my head this time, it was down by my side.

When I happened to feel my armpit again a few weeks later whilst lying in bed, again with my arm above my head, the lump was back. Well, it had never gone away; I just couldn't feel it with my arm down by my side.

I decided that I ought to get this out-of-place lump checked, so I went to my GP. Knowing the links between an armpit lump and breast cancer, the GP examined my breasts. I'm no stranger to having my breasts checked. I have lumpy boobs. Perfectly harmless cysts. They arrived around four years ago and I was told, "Well, it's just something that women of your age get. Nothing to worry about. No increased risk of developing breast cancer. Just innocent little pockets of liquid."

Upon her examination, the GP could only feel my existing, squishy breast cysts and no hard, worrying lumps, nor any other signs that something was seriously amiss. She didn't quite know what to make of it, so she suggested that I get myself checked out at the hospital breast clinic.

Following my visit to the GP, I wasn't overly concerned by this armpit lump. I just assumed that it was a cyst, but in my armpit instead of my breast. I was due to have one of my regular cyst check-ups at the breast clinic anyway, so on the GP's suggestion, I duly made an appointment.

The appointment was when my husband happened to be away for a week with his new job. I was so confident that the lump was nothing to worry about that I didn't even tell my husband I was going to the hospital. I thought that, given the past four years' worth of uneventful breast clinic appointments, this one would be no different and I needn't worry him unnecessarily whilst he was away.

The day of the appointment arrived and I turned up at the clinic. In the changing area I took off my top and bra and put on a threadbare hospital gown, which I then covered with a washed-out hospital robe. I was told to keep my jeans and boots on: it was a strange look, but no one was judging. I then calmly waited for my appointment in the waiting room with all the other women in their jeans and boots, gowns and robes.

First up was a mammogram, which consisted of standing topless in a freezing cold room, where each breast was squished and squashed into a large whirring machine; a bit like squeezing each boob into a flat sandwich toaster. Just when you think the squeezing has reached a point where the boob cannot be squeezed any further, it squeezes just a little further and then it's over.

I had to sit in the waiting room a little while longer before being called in to see the breast consultant.

"Mrs Lee... Lee... Lee-ann-arge?"

Nobody ever pronounces my surname properly the first time round.

"Yes."

"Come through now, please."

I went into the breast consultant's room. There was the standard hospital desk, beside which sat Mr Breast Consultant on one of the three hospital chairs. Mr Breast Consultant is old and wise, maybe late sixties with white hair and a small hearing aid. He has a very kind face and a reassuring manner.

As with every other time I'd been to see him to have my breast cysts checked, I felt like a bit of a fraud as I sat facing him, on one of the other chairs. There I was, taking up an important man's valuable time with my innocent little pockets of liquid, while other women waiting to see him may well have some not-so-innocent little lumps. He'd always told me that I must try to see him once a year or so, because I wouldn't be able to tell the difference between a cyst and 'something else' (by which I always assumed he meant cancerous lump but didn't want to worry me by saying those words). So, there I was, sitting on a hard, plastic chair across the desk from his expectant gaze.

"I've found a lump in my armpit and because it was about time for you to check out my cysts here I am but I'm not worried about the lump because I found it in August on holiday but then I lost it and couldn't feel it but then I found it again," I waffled without taking a breath.

Somehow or other, sitting in that chair in the breast clinic made me feel a little bit on edge.

"Right, let's get you up on the couch and take a look then."

I knew the routine. I took off the gown and robe and sat sideways on the high couch, naked from the waist up, with Mr Breast Consultant facing me, a few feet back and crouching down so that his eyes were level with my breasts.

"Arms down by your sides, please."

Ten seconds of intent staring passed.

"Arms above your head, please."

Another ten seconds of intent staring passed.

"Lie down now, please."

And with that, he started his routine of pressing, prodding and pushing my boobs, neck and armpits whilst raising and lowering my arms. As always, I turned my head to the side so as to avoid awkward eye contact with this man I hardly knew who was having a good feel of my breasts. Yes, I had been through this examination a number of times before, but that didn't make the experience any less uncomfortable.

I remember being mortified when I went through it for the first time four years ago. It is completely and utterly contrary to normal behaviour, to be bare chested in front of strangers, let alone someone who stares, then proceeds to have a good grope. For me, my chest area is personal, private and secret: closed to everyone. On the other hand, to Mr Breast Consultant, my chest area is merely part of the anatomy requiring investigation because something is not quite right.

Mr Breast Consultant pulled out his marker pen and drew a few squiggles over both breasts: a road map for the ultrasound radiographer to check out a few new lumps (a.k.a. suspected cysts). Again, I wasn't worried at this point. It was normal practice to which I'd become accustomed over the years. He indicated that he couldn't find anything of concern in either breast, just a few new cysts and, as such, he wasn't worried about the armpit lump—it was probably a blocked gland.

"You can get dressed now," Mr Breast Consultant said, with his back to me as he washed his hands.

Linda, the nurse who'd been in the room the whole time, helped me back into my gown and robe whilst chatting to me about something normal and mundane; probably the weather.

"Well, I don't think there's anything to worry about, but we'll do an ultrasound now just to make sure," he said.

Again, nothing to worry about. All normal practice.

I'd had ultrasound scans on my breasts before. I knew what to expect. As usual, the radiographer sat at a computer next to a couch on which I lay, again topless. Then she covered what looked like a microphone in cold lubricant jelly and pressed this lubricated microphone over my breasts, following Mr Breast Consultant's road map of marker-pen scribbles. She looked at the computer screen most of the time, pressing buttons to snap black-and-white images of the insides of my lumpy breasts.

On this occasion I had a fairly chatty radiographer who gave me a running commentary about each of the cysts: their size, shape and whether it would be worth aspirating them to make them less uncomfortable for me.

Then, she came to the armpit lump. It didn't look like the breast lumps on her computer screen and she suggested a biopsy just to "cover all bases." Now, I'd never had a biopsy of any of my breast lumps, so when she pulled out the biggest needle I'd ever seen, I must have gone completely white. I hate, hate, hate needles! Especially when they are going into me.

The procedure was painful and uncomfortable. It was quite tricky for the radiographer to reach across me (still topless) and insert the needle into the teeny tiny lump in my armpit whilst using the lubricated microphone to establish the location of said lump as she looked at her computer screen. Being the wimp I am, I was decidedly shaken by the whole procedure. Not out of fear of what the test might find, but because I'd had a huge needle stuck into my armpit!

After more waiting around with all the other gowned, robed and worried-looking ladies, I went back in to see Mr Breast Consultant. He'd had a chance to look at the mammogram and the ultrasound images. He didn't seem the least bit concerned. There were no suspicious lumps showing up in my breasts from either scan. He sent me on my way and told me to come back in a week's time for the results of the biopsy.

As Linda showed me out, she said, "When you come back for the results, you might want to bring someone with you."

I wasn't overly concerned. I certainly didn't think that breast cancer was on the cards because both breast scans had been clear. I'm no medical expert but I knew that the worst case scenario of breast cancer was unlikely, if not impossible. I didn't have a suspicious lump in either breast, or any of the other tell-tale signs of breast cancer. No inverted nipples, dimpling, discharge, pain or reddening skin (plus, I was only forty-two and ticked all the boxes on the list of things to do to reduce the risk of cancer, being the young, non-smoking, exercising, healthy woman with no family history of cancer that I am).

Life continued as normal following the biopsy. My husband was back from his trip and we had the usual:

1. Work.
2. School.
3. Kids' activities.
4. Homework.
5. Never ending to-do list tasks.
6. Life admin.

We did have a particularly nice weekend though: my cousin Kate and her family came to stay for the weekend. We chatted, we walked, we ate, we drank and we sang Eighties and Nineties songs at the tops of our lungs way into the night without a care in the world.

A few weeks earlier, my husband found a bottle of wine in the cupboard that we'd been given as a wedding present. We've been married just over thirteen years. It had been hiding from us all that time. We drank it that weekend with Kate and her husband, Stuart. We smugly toasted marriage, kids and how well we had all done over the past thirteen years. Life was good. Pretty great actually.

My follow-up appointment was on a Wednesday evening. Given the timing of the appointment, I went to work as normal that day. I'm a solicitor. Before I had children, I worked long hours, the odd weekend and had dreams of travel, success and partnership.

Then I had children and my priorities changed. I wanted to be around for them, pick them up from school, make their tea and be as much of a hands-on mum as possible. Of course, I also wanted the career, so I had to make some adjustments and compromise on both counts. I took a pay cut, reduced my hours and became a professional support lawyer; out went all dreams of travel, success and partnership.

Instead of working for clients, I started working for my team, organising training, monitoring legal developments and developing the business. It's interesting, engaging and challenging. Now, I have two jobs: full-time mum and part-time (but sometimes feels like full-time) lawyer. At times it's crazily busy, but I'm not complaining. I'm happy with both.

As I went to leave the office at the end of the day, I had my usual short parting chat with two of the PAs who I've known for years and who I absolutely adore. Working with the same people in the same office day after day, year after year, creates a special bond. I've known Debbie and Sandra for longer than I've known many of my friends. They are like my big sisters. I'll bend their ears, cry on their shoulders and moan with them until the cows come home.

"So, anything nice this evening, Sara?"

"Mmm, not really. I have an appointment with the breast consultant."

"The usual?"

They are, of course, fully aware of my breast cyst situation as much as every other personal situation that I have ever experienced.

"Err, I'm not sure. It's the results of a biopsy on a lump in my armpit this time. It's probably just the same thing as the other cysts. Just a bit weird that I had to have it tested. Anyway, I've been here before, needlessly worrying, so I'm sure it'll be fine."

It didn't quite work out like that, though.

Heeding the words of lovely nurse Linda, my mum came with me to the appointment. My husband wasn't due home from work until later in the evening and given my lack of concern, it didn't seem necessary for him to get home early to come with me.

When we arrived at the hospital, we were told to wait in a different waiting room to the one in which the gowned and robed ladies sat. In hindsight, that should have alerted me to the fact that something was off.

We didn't have to wait long until we were called in to see Mr Breast Consultant in his familiar room. Linda wasn't there; in her place was an unfamiliar face. Mr Breast Consultant introduced her as Amber, the hospital breast care nurse, but before I'd had time to fully process the presence of a breast care nurse at this appointment, we were sitting down and Mr Breast Consultant was delivering The News.

"I'm afraid it's not good news. We've found cancer cells in your lymph nodes."

BAM.

With that, the air in the room was sucked out. I couldn't catch my breath. I froze in my chair and my entire body started to shake. I'd never experienced shaking from shock before. I thought it was just a saying or something that happened on the television or in films. I didn't cry, nor make any noise: no low moaning, howling or screaming. I couldn't speak. My brain just couldn't work out what to say at that point.

Mum took over and broke the silence. She sat up very straight in her plastic chair, held up her chin and started speaking. I remember turning to look at her face.

She wasn't crying, which surprised me because my mum is a huge softie and it's not unusual for her to cry at the smallest thing, let alone at the news that her daughter has cancer. Instead, there was my straight-backed, incredibly brave mum asking all the questions I should've been asking but couldn't because my brain, mouth, body connections had gone horribly wrong.

I hadn't been expecting him to tell me that I had cancer. That just wasn't an outcome for which I was prepared, and I was unprepared in more ways than one.

I didn't have one of my pencils, nor any paper on which to take notes: diagnosis details, stage and grade of cancer, surgery options and next steps.

I'd fumbled in my bag with my shaking hands to double check I didn't have a pencil and piece of paper. I felt that finding them would bring some normality to this entirely abnormal situation. Under normal circumstances it would have been precisely the type of situation in which I would be writing down every word, ready to go home and research my options.

You see, I am very good at life projects. Yes, I am one of those people who some might call boringly organised and lacking in spontaneity. I take all the available information, read up on the subject, note down tips and advice, prepare to-do lists, then embark upon the project with vigour, ploughing ahead with all the information I can locate.

Whether it's a big project like organising my wedding, planning a home extension, or something a little less consequential like booking a holiday, putting on a birthday party or ordering a new washing machine, my approach to life projects tends to follow the same pattern:

1. Research the situation.
2. Investigate the options.
3. Note down the choices.
4. Write a plan of how to proceed.
5. Put the plan into action.

On this particular day I wasn't expecting to be starting Project Breast Cancer. I was expecting Mr Breast Consultant to tell me that the hard, marble-sized ball in my left armpit was a harmless cyst, or blocked node, or swollen gland, or something similar.

He didn't tell me that. What he did tell me was, "We've found cancer cells in your lymph nodes. We think it's breast cancer."

After what felt like hours sitting in the hot, stuffy consulting room, during which Mum and Mr Breast Consultant talked about the diagnosis, Amber walked us out. She handed over a booklet and some leaflets while she explained, in her calming voice, the next steps. I couldn't focus on what she was saying. She had a friendly face and kind eyes. Her mouth was moving and she had a lovely voice, but what she was saying didn't make any sense to me.

My brain had exploded and I could not return to rational thinking. Understanding the state of shock that I was in, Amber addressed my mum and I let them discuss what would happen from now on and then make arrangements for the next appointment.

I was vaguely aware of the hospital humdrum continuing around me; everything was exactly as it had been when I walked into the hospital earlier that evening, and yet everything was completely different. I felt like I'd been transported out of normal life and thrown into an entirely different, unfamiliar place.

The calm, serene waiting room looked the same and yet it now felt horribly oppressive. The busy buzz of the hospital now felt depressing. The constant hospital din of patient voices, lifts pinging, doors opening and nurses shouting was muffled as if I were underwater.

Not only was my brain not working properly, but other parts of my body didn't want to function. I was walking through treacle; my feet wouldn't move as fast as I wanted them to. My shaking hands struggled to button up my coat and I ended up just wrapping it around me, maybe subconsciously trying to hold myself up at the same time.

I had to focus on breathing—moving my chest up then down to take air into my lungs—because the process of breathing on autopilot didn't seem to be working properly.

Yet, somehow or other, I made it out of the hospital that evening, and I made it through the subsequent twelve days.

CHECKLIST

Tips For Attending Your Medical Appointments

- Take someone with you. Not only will they provide moral support, but they will also be able to help you remember what the doctors tell you. It can be hard to remember everything at this time because there's a lot to take in and you may well be in a state of shock.
- Take a notebook and pen so that your companion can make a note of everything that's discussed during the appointment. You can read this at home when you are feeling calmer.
- Make a note of any questions/concerns that you have as and when you think of them between appointments, because you may forget them if you are still processing your diagnosis.
- Go to each appointment prepared with your list of questions.
- If in doubt about anything, ask.

CHAPTER 4

I DON'T LIKE A 'BUT'

*"A strong woman looks a challenge dead in the eye
and gives it a wink."*
Gina Carey

I'm still here at the kitchen table staring at the remains of lunch, not yet able to summon the energy to clear the plates. Thinking about one's own cancer diagnosis is incredibly draining.

The children are in the lounge watching Halloween cartoons on the TV, without a care in the world other than wondering how many sweets they'll bring home this evening.

When Mr Breast Consultant told me, at the D-Day appointment, that they'd found what they thought were breast cancer cells in my lymph nodes, I remember thinking, but not being able to articulate out loud: *What do you mean you think it's breast cancer? How can you not be sure?*

It was bad enough to be told that cancer cells had been found in my lymph nodes, but then to be told that they were not entirely sure where the cancer cells had come from was doubly, triply scary. I mean, surely breast cancer cells come from, well, a breast? It's all there in the name of this type of cancer!

Thanks to Mum, who took great care in remembering every

single word that was said at the D-Day appointment, what they *did* know for certain was:

1. The biopsy of the lump in my armpit had tested positive for cancer.
2. The lump was a collection of cancer cells in my lymph nodes.
3. The markings on these cells indicated that it was breast cancer but the mammogram and ultrasound had shown no signs of a tumour in either breast.
4. I would need to be checked from head to toe by a variety of scans to see if (a) a tumour could be found in either breast, which had not been picked up by the mammogram or ultrasound, and/or (b) a tumour could be located anywhere else within me.

Of course, this uncertainty surrounding the origination of the cancer cells caused me a fair amount of worry, heart-stopping panic and confusion. If I had stray cancer cells appearing in my lymph nodes, where had they come from? Where else could they be?

A number of possible explanations raced around my mind during the days following D-Day. Given that I have absolutely no medical background, nor any experience of being close to someone who has gone through breast cancer, the possibilities were over exaggerated, worst case scenario and, it turns out, ultimately wrong. However, I was thankfully unable to wallow around in blind anguish for too long because the first scan was scheduled to take place within a few days.

On a grey, dismal October morning, while I was feeling

as gloomy as the weather, I had a boob MRI. I'm not a fan of MRIs at the best of times—it's the scan with the long, narrow tube. You have to lie on a table and are inserted into the tube and left alone in there while the radiographers go off to another room to fiddle with dials, controls and computers.

The nurses kindly offer you headphones and a choice of music (classical please, to help soothe me) but there's no point to the music because all you can hear is the extremely loud pounding of the magnets, booming, clanking and hammering.

I'm slightly claustrophobic. I would rather take the stairs than the lift. I don't like going on the London Underground. I would never ever in a million years go caving (I feel shaky just thinking about that) and the thought of being inserted into a tube and left all alone makes me break out in sweat, but I decided to be brave for the boob MRI.

I knew that it was going to be the first in a long line of scans and tests, let alone whatever challenges the cancer treatment would bring. So, I made the decision to try to get over my claustrophobia and just get on with it.

Mum insisted on taking me back to the hospital for the MRI. She and Dad said there'd be plenty of times when my husband would need to accompany me to important consultant appointments and treatment sessions, so to minimise the need for time off his new job they would help out with the scan appointments.

This worked well for me and my husband. He was aware that he'd need time off over the coming months, and I'd regressed to being a daughter in need of parental care and comfort.

When we arrived at the Diagnostic Imaging department of the hospital I had to leave Mum in the main waiting room and go into the MRI room on my own. Without either of us saying anything, I knew that neither of us were particularly happy about this. Me with my reinforced, childlike-need for hand holding and Mum with her maternal instincts kicking in at full throttle.

Holding up my chin, I went in on my own. I changed into the familiar hospital gown. I had to leave the opening at the front this time, not at the back, which caused much gaping. I just had my knickers on underneath. Big, grey, washed-out granny pants, which were a bad choice for that day. My knicker drawer was empty that morning because I hadn't had the focus to do any washing for the past few days. My socks were mismatched.

Under usual circumstances that would have thrown me off kilter for the day, but circumstances were far from usual. Everything felt rather surreal as I sat, fussing with the gaping, threadbare gown, waiting for my turn.

A nurse came over to me to insert a cannula into my left inner elbow, through which they were planning to pump some purple dye midway through the scan to help with imaging the breast tissue.

A cannula is basically a needle going into a vein, with plastic casing on the end, allowing it to be hooked up to an intravenous drip, syringe or something similar. Well, needing a cannula was not expected. Not expected at all, so I hadn't prepared myself for it.

The memory of the biopsy needle was still fresh in my mind, but I realised that this was only the tip of the needle iceberg, and my immediate future held numerous situations where I was to expect needles. Again, I decided to get over my fears and be brave. I took a deep breath and in went the cannula.

It was decidedly uncomfortable because I was then unable to bend that elbow; it's only when you know that you cannot bend your elbow that you oh so desperately need to bend that elbow!

I had a little while to wait, sitting in a chair in the waiting area in my mis-matched socks and gaping gown with my unbending elbow, waiting to be inserted into the long, narrow tube all alone. I really was trying to be brave. I bit my lip. I took a few deep breaths. I tried to think of anything other than what I was doing right then, and anything other than cancer and all the fear that the diagnosis had brought me.

My brave face clearly wasn't convincing because a lovely nurse, Sharon (to whom I owe a lot because she subsequently held my hand through many scans and hugs me every time she now sees me in the hospital) came over to me and tried to make me feel more at ease. As her opener, she asked me about my children. Well, that was it. The floodgates opened and I couldn't hold the tears back. My chin crumpled and my bottom lip gave way. Tissues were handed over. Shoulders were patted. Soothing words were spoken. I eventually managed to calm myself down, ready to enter the room for my session in the tube.

Walking into the scanning room itself, the first thing I saw was a narrow trolley table with two holes positioned just under a forehead rest. No need to guess what they were for: yes, obviously my boobs. The holes were on the large size, clearly for the ample-bosomed lady; mine were going to be lost in there! As I looked at the boob holes, I realised that I was going to have to lie down on my front on the trolley table, which posed a slight problem because I have a bad back. I can't easily lie on my front because my spine sort of fuses into a stiff, unbending, immoveable rod and I cannot easily get up again.

With a feeling of rising despair, I realised that I was going to have to climb up onto the trolley table without bending my left arm (because it had a freaking needle in it) and I was going to have to open my gown and insert my boobs into the holes without bending my left arm (because it had a freaking needle in it). I would need to lie myself down with my dodgy back twinging, all the while without bending my left arm. I would then be left in the long, dark, narrow, teeny tiny tube all on my own for thirty minutes and, oh my, I would need to reverse the whole procedure at the end of the scan.

Not only was I worried about actually getting on and off the table, I also wanted to do all this without flashing my boobs or my big, grey, washed-out granny pants.

You know those two wonderfully subtle traits we grab hold of in times of stress to help get us through it and out the other side—grace and dignity? Well, grace and dignity most definitely flew out the window the moment I entered the scan room. It wasn't a pretty sight. Boobs were definitely flashed and granny pants were most certainly on full view, as I contorted into all sorts of positions to get onto the table and then off the table, whilst trying to minimise pain to my back and without bending my arm. Let's just say that everyone was very nice about it.

A few days after the MRI, my husband and I went to see Mr Breast Consultant, hopeful that the sensitive and invasive MRI had been able to locate what the mammogram and ultrasound had been unable to detect: a tumour in one of my breasts. We were hopeful because if there was a lump in a breast then we would know exactly what we were dealing with. We'd be able to move on and sort it all out, and my mind could stop playing games with me, teasing me about the alternative explanations.

Unfortunately, the MRI couldn't locate a tumour in either breast, so onwards (but not upwards) and I was booked in for something called a CT PET scan to see if there was a tumour somewhere else inside me.

This was at a different hospital, about forty-five minutes away by car, and this time Dad offered to drive me and wait while I had the scan and drive me home again.

My dad is always there for my sister and me. I know I could call him at three in the morning from five hundred miles away and he would come to the rescue (albeit he might be a tad grumpy). He never shows his feelings or talks about his worries. He's not an emotional man, he's a practical man: one typical of his generation.

When I was diagnosed, Dad and Mum were planning a holiday. He'd said to her, "Well, that's it, Jen, we're just going to have to drop everything for the foreseeable future."

It made my heart swell when I heard he'd said that but my heart also ached for them. Nobody wants to watch their child (even a grown-up child) go through cancer and nobody wants to cancel a holiday.

Whilst this next scan did not involve boob holes or a long, dark tube, it brought its own challenges. This was my first visit to a large cancer-focused hospital. When Dad and I walked in, we were greeted by the cancer information desk. There were so many booklets and information packs about every type of cancer. I was hit by a wall of informational posters and leaflets showing bald men and bald women with cups of tea, talking to nurses, walking on beaches, gardening and holding hands with their significant others.

I felt all of them gazing down at me from the posters and leaflets with the knowing look of people who've been travelling along some sort of cancer road for a while, watching with pity as newly diagnosed me walked past them amidst an air of confusion, uncertainty and cancer naivety.

In the few seconds it took us to walk past the information desk, a wave of realisation washed over me. *I have cancer. I am in a cancer hospital. With other cancer people. People with cancer. Cancer patients. Oh shit! I'm a cancer patient.*

Dad and I (the rather wobbly, decidedly scared, trying-to-be-brave cancer patient) made our way through the maze of corridors to the scanning department, where we then had to wait for a long time with other people who were also waiting for their scans.

There were no bald people in that waiting room. All at the start of the road like me. Perhaps not even at the start of a cancer road, but some other road. None of us looked ill. We were just a bunch of normal looking people waiting for tests to show our not so normalness. Nobody was catching the eye of anyone else. Magazines and newspapers were being stared at but not read.

The people who were being called for the more routine type of scan, like CT scans and MRIs, were being taken down the corridor straight ahead, whilst those patients having the radioactive CT PET scan had to go through a special door to the right, with a special lock requiring a special code and special nurses in special clothes. I was finally called in for my special scan. I was not feeling special.

Dad waved me off and I entered the wing. Alone again. It was all very clinical and hospital-ish and scary, but again it was time to be brave. I knew that hospitals and scans were going to be my life for the foreseeable future so I had to pull myself together and deal with it but I was about to be injected with a radioactive isotope. I was feeling far from brave. I tried to console myself with the fact that at least there wouldn't be a long, narrow, dark tube to lie in this time.

The radiographer who called me in was around my age, possibly a little bit older. She looked serious, mature and kind, and she looked like she knew what she was doing, which was, of course, a good sign because radioactivity was involved.

Once again, I wasn't sure that my brave face showed, because she talked to me slowly and calmly, as if I were either a child or incredibly old. I didn't mind. She explained the procedure and got me ready with my inner elbow cannula, which was all very familiar. Unlike the MRI, I was going to be injected before the scan and not during it, so I wouldn't need to have the cannula in place during the scan and I could bend my elbow left, right and centre if I wanted to.

There was also no need to change out of my clothes and into a gown this time, which was wonderful news given that I was at the very bottom of the knicker drawer that day.

Just as I was lulled into a false sense of 'this is actually going to be alright,' she wheeled in a metal trolley and things got a bit weird (and, well, I suppose it explained the special door, special lock, special code and special nurses).

On top of the trolley was a small metal canister, the size of a Big Mac box. The radiographer put on a very heavy-duty apron and opened the metal canister. I'd like to say she opened the metal canister with a whoosh and that steam poured out of it, but I think that would be my imagination and not a true recollection of events.

Then we got to the bit where I thought that I was in some sort of sci-fi film. Inside the metal Big Mac canister was a little vial, which she took out with giant tweezers. In hindsight, I am surprised that the radiographer was not in a full hazmat suit. This was the radioactive isotope that was going to be injected into me.

INTO. ME.

With all the fanfare of wheeling in and opening the metal Big Mac canister (plus the whooshing and steam in my mind's eye), I barely noticed the actual injection into my cannula. I had officially become Radioactive Girl.

It takes a while for a radioactive isotope to make its way around every part of your insides, so I had to lie down on a hard, narrow bed behind a curtain for half an hour, very, very still. I couldn't move. I don't know why, but those were the instructions, and as someone who faithfully follows instructions and rules, I lay completely still until I was collected by a nurse for the scan itself.

Whilst waiting on the bed, I could see part of a clock through a gap between the curtains. Not the half with the hands, so it didn't help me to pass the time. I could also see a lady in a wheelchair. She was asleep with her head slumped back, mouth open and snoring. I was glad she was snoring because that's how I knew she was alive.

She was very thin and sallow, and her clothes were hanging off her. She was hooked up to an IV. At first, I thought that she was an elderly lady, maybe in her seventies or eighties, but as I had a good half hour to stare at her, I realised that she wasn't actually all that old.

She was older than me, but possibly only by ten years, rather than thirty or so. It was sad how comfortable she looked in her wheelchair with her IV, as if she'd been side by side with her IV for some time. She was wheeled away and I couldn't help but relate myself to her. *Would I, at some point down the line, become the snoring woman in the wheelchair?*

Then it was my turn to be scanned. It was fine. It was not uncomfortable. It was not unpleasant. It was just lying on a table, which had a giant plastic donut around it. The donut moved up and down the table, making whirring noises as it did its job of looking inside me, seeking out the radioactivity and seeking out the place within me that had gone wrong. I felt smug. I could deal with these scans, thank you very much.

When it was over I was taken back to my narrow bed behind the curtain where I waited for a little while longer, presumably so they could check I didn't have an adverse reaction to the isotope and to allow the radioactivity to disperse some more before I was let out into the real world. Finally, I was allowed to leave.

The nurses kindly called out for my dad who'd calmly, patiently, lovingly, uncomplainingly and voluntarily waited for four hours while his eldest daughter had been scanned for signs of where her cancer had originated. He is a saint. I was radioactive. I could not go within one metre of him, or anyone else for that matter. It was in the instructions and I had to follow those to the letter.

The drive home was interesting. I sat in the back seat on

the other side of the car from Dad, and I wedged myself as close to the door as I could, trying to put as much distance as I could between me and Dad.

Forty-five minutes or so later, we arrived home to an empty house because my mum had collected the children from school and taken them home for the night, keeping them away from their radioactive mother who wasn't allowed near them for twelve hours.

Dad settled me onto the sofa, taking care not to come within the fallout zone of one metre. Then off he went and I was left alone. Again.

I needed a hug. I needed some comfort. I needed someone to tell me that everything was going to be alright. I needed to not be alone. So, when my husband came home from work and walked into the lounge where I was positioned on the sofa feeling sorry for myself, I just wanted him to wrap me in his arms where I would feel safe and protected. I wanted him to hug me and tell me we would get through this but there was that bloody one-metre fallout zone.

He sat as close to me as he was allowed, and we stared at, rather than watched, whatever programme happened to be on the TV, each of us probably lost in our own worries about what the CT PET scan would show.

The CT PET scan is apparently the holy grail of all scans. It is ultra-sensitive and can pick up anything inside someone that is not as it should be. All hopes were on this scan pinpointing the source of those stray cancer cells in my armpit.

The results had arrived on Mr Breast Consultant's desk, so my husband, my new 'Project Cancer Notebook' and I went off to see him. I may have been completely unprepared for the D-Day appointment but that wasn't going to happen again.

Within a few days of D-Day, I had got some (not much) of my organisational mojo back and I had organised Project Cancer Notebook. Unfortunately, due to a combination of time constraints and my mind not really being up to anything other than worrying about what was going on, I didn't buy a new, shiny, pretty notebook. Instead, I chose an already partly used, rather dog-eared notebook that I'd found during a quick rummage through my daughter's bedroom.

After tearing out the used pages and marking the front with my name in a sharpie (I couldn't face writing down the word 'cancer'), Project Cancer Notebook was ready to go.

My husband was appointed guardian of the Project Cancer Notebook because I had sat through every appointment up to that point, completely paralysed from head to toe, unable to comprehend what was going on. He, on the other hand, was being super attentive and was still able to think straight.

We went into the familiar consulting room and I knew even before Mr Breast Consultant had finished his opening sentence that there was a 'but' coming.

"Well, the CT PET scan and the blood tests have ruled out cancer in the bowel, bones, brain, ovaries, lungs, cervix and stomach. But it did show a little shadow on the pancreas and also one on the thyroid, so I'd like to arrange a pancreatic MRI and thyroid scan."

I couldn't sit still in my chair. My legs were fidgeting and twitching. I felt very hot. I needed some air. I was struggling to focus on what was being said.

Mr Breast Consultant was talking to my husband who was

asking questions and writing things down in Project Cancer Notebook and then they looked at me. Was I meant to say something? Answer a question?

"You don't look very happy," observed Mr Breast Consultant. "You should do because it's good news. We've ruled out cancer in a number of places, and we just need to check these shadows to rule out the possibility of cancer in the thyroid and pancreas." He gave me a quizzical glance.

"I don't like the but," I said. I felt like a spoilt, complaining child.

Mr Breast Consultant was being, as usual, very calm and very nice. His white hair indicated that he'd been in this game for quite a few years and knew what he was talking about. Even so, I was the one who had to go home no closer to knowing what was going on inside me and hence where I was going to end up.

I'd had high hopes that during that appointment with Mr Breast Consultant we would have found out the source of the evil cancer cells and we could at least move forward in getting rid of them and getting me back to *me*. I felt that all my hopes had been dashed, new worries had been put on the table and I was getting really confused because if the cancer cells showed markings of breast cancer, why would they be looking at my pancreas and thyroid? And he was talking about me having another dreadful MRI.

So, it was back to the Diagnostic Imaging department of my usual hospital for another MRI. Sharon, the lovely nurse, was there again and I felt like we were old friends as she hugged me when I walked in. I felt like an old pro when it came to the scan. It was a repeat of the boob MRI with a few tweaks. No booby holes though, and this time I had to lie on my back, which was much easier for maintaining dignity where the gown was concerned.

The cannula was put in place with dye ready to be injected midway through the scan. There was the clanking and clinking of the magnets, the headphones and the drowned-out music. There was the long, narrow tube. Again, I tried to be brave, following the instructions of when to breathe in and when to breathe out.

With this being the third scan involving some sort of claustrophobic body tube or donut, I'd given some thought as to how best to get through the scan bit—the lying-in-the-tube-all-alone bit. I realised that I needed some sort of mental distraction, something that would require brain power and from which it would be harder to be distracted.

Having spent quite a lot of the past few years practising times tables with my children in the car on the way to school, I decided to give them a go. In my mind, I said them slowly and in full. I started with *one times two equals two*, moved on to *two times two equals four* and carried on all the way up to the twelve times tables. I even tried to use the tempo of the clanking magnets to get a rhythm going and it worked. I was so busy with my childhood maths recital that the scan was over before I'd even been through the entire repertoire three times.

A few days later, it was time for what I hoped would be the final scan; one of my thyroid. Thankfully, that scan did not involve any giant tubes or giant donuts. It was just a little ultrasound on my neck—very similar to the original breast ultrasound, but happily I didn't need to go topless.

My friend Gina took me to the hospital for that one. By

this point, I'd told a few close friends about what was going on. Partly because I needed some support from my best friends. Partly because I needed help with childcare whilst I was to-ing and fro-ing from all the hospital appointments. Partly because sometimes I just couldn't mask the I-have-just-found-out-that-my-world-is-falling-apart look.

Gina was allowed to come into the consulting room for the duration of the ultrasound, which made a nice change from being alone during the previous scans. We were chatting about my cancer fears as we waited for the consultant to come in and start work on me.

"I'm still not quite sure why they think cancer could be in my thyroid and pancreas."

"Well, I suppose it's more to rule out all other possible reasons for the cancer cells being in your lymph nodes," Gina said trying to reassure me.

She was right, of course. That was exactly why I was getting my pancreas and thyroid checked out—they were ruling out everything that could possibly be ruled out.

There was a nurse in the room who overheard our conversation and she joined in. Because, it turned out, she had recently finished treatment for breast cancer and she looked amazingly normal (I know that doesn't sound right, but when everything is just getting more and more abnormal, something normal can be amazing). Plus, she was working.

She didn't look in any way like she'd been ill, let alone had treatment for cancer. Unlike the people on the posters and leaflets at the cancer centre, she had hair. Proper, real, normal hair. She'd had cancer, she'd had treatment, she was back at work and she looked fabulous.

I'm thinking about that nurse as I sit here now, at my kitchen table with the remnants of lunch still not cleared away. I wonder whether I'll be like that nurse who went through hell and came out the other side. After the rollercoaster of the past few weeks, I wonder what's in store for me next.

The list of appointments that I've had so far looks like this:

1. Mammogram.
2. Ultrasound.
3. Cancer diagnosis.
4. Booby MRI.
5. Follow-up consultant appointment.
6. CT PET.
7. Another follow-up consultant appointment.
8. Pancreatic MRI.
9. Thyroid ultrasound.

I've got my next appointment with Mr Breast Consultant the day after tomorrow. I'm desperately hoping that Mr Breast Consultant will have some answers to the conundrum that is my cancer because, maybe, once we establish exactly what we're dealing with, I can look it hard and straight in the eye, and maybe I can get through it and come out the other side, just like the nurse. But today is my daughter's favourite day of the year. Let's clear this table and get cracking with Halloween.

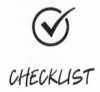

CHECKLIST

Scans

- Get used to baring your breasts, they are not boobs/boobies/knockers to the medical team, rather just part of your anatomy that needs to be checked and investigated.
- Ask someone to take you so that you don't have to drive yourself. Company is also an excellent distraction from any fears you may have about the scans themselves and the diagnosis.
- Nobody cares what underwear you're wearing.
- Some of the machines can look big, scary and sometimes plain weird but the scans are over pretty quickly and they don't hurt.
- Be prepared to be cold! The machinery has to be kept at a certain temperature so it is usually cold in the scan rooms—ask for a blanket.
- To eat or not to eat? Before you go, follow any instructions that you've been given about fasting. Sometimes you're injected with a dye so that they can see your organs and you're not allowed to eat or drink for a certain time beforehand.

- Nurses and radiographers are usually very kind and understanding. Tell them if you're uncertain about the procedure.
- Don't be afraid to ask questions. Take a notebook and pen in which you have jotted down your questions, and you can write any notes.
- Take your mind off what is going on during the scan by distracting yourself with a mind game or relaxation technique. Times tables are a good one.
- The waiting game. If you have to wait for results and you haven't heard by when you had expected, there is no harm in calling up for the results.

If you want to learn more about the different types of scans you can look at the Cancer Research UK website (see Appendix).

CHAPTER 5

WELLIES, HOT CHOCOLATE, WARM JUMPERS AND COLD NOSES

"Life is tough my darling, but so are you."
Stephanie Bennett-Henry

We're at the next date in the autumn calendar: Bonfire Night. I usually like autumn because I love the colours of the changing leaves, the sound of rain pounding against the windows, the musty smell of conkers mixed with mouldy leaves, and the low sunshine.

I love it when the season changes from summer to autumn, so we can officially give up hoping for warm weather that isn't coming and just accept the grey dampness of the English climate. I love snuggling up indoors under soft blankets because, at heart, I suppose I am a homely girl.

I know that most people think of spring as the season of change, but for me autumn has always represented a turning point. An 'out with the old, in with the new' phase: a new term at school, the changing weather and the promise of cosy evenings at home.

However, autumn this year does not hold the same promises for me. I feel that autumn marks the end of something good and nice. That we are moving from something bright and carefree to something dull and gloomy. That the loss of leaves from the trees is not making way for fresh new buds next spring, but rather marks the loss of something special, unique and important, leaving them barren, forlorn and sad.

Nonetheless, it's Bonfire Night. I usually like standing in the middle of a dark field wrapped up in warm layers, wellies and warm socks, holding a polystyrene cup of something hot to drink. I like the buzz of the crowd milling around the huge bonfire in anticipation of the fireworks. I love watching the children running around with their friends, excited to be out and left to their own devices and that at the end of the fireworks, we go back to the car with cold hands and noses to drink mugs of hot chocolate whilst the kids and their friends pile into the boot of the car, with their wellies and coats flung off.

However, tonight, I'm not really in the mood. I don't want to see people and make small talk and paste on a smile and pretend that everything is fine. I'm not in the mood to listen to other people talk about insignificant, immaterial, petty trivialities. Because, quite frankly, right now, unless someone has cancer and talks to me about that, I'm afraid that whatever they have to say will seem like insignificant, immaterial, petty trivialities. I'm feeling grumpy and really rather sorry for myself.

I'm now two and a half weeks into my cancer diagnosis and I've spent it being scanned, injected, poked, prodded and tested. I've hardly eaten a thing and I'm pretty sure I haven't slept. I feel like a completely different person to the one who woke up on the morning of October 19th, blissfully unaware of what was to unfold from that day onwards.

For the past two and half weeks I've avoided seeing anyone

other than my family and a few close friends. No matter how hard I try, I just can't turn off the cancer switch in my brain. It's all I can think about. I've lost the ability to be 'normal.' Whilst I don't look like I have cancer, I feel like the word is tattooed across my forehead. So, tonight is a bit of a big deal for me—having to camouflage the 'cancer tattoo' and put on my public face.

I expect to deal with this evening in one of two ways. I will either find the courage to just go about the evening as if it's any other normal, non-cancer, nothing-to-do-with-cancer evening. Or I will cower and hide and hope that I don't cross paths with anyone I even vaguely know, for fear that they may see through me and know that something is not quite right.

On Wednesday, my husband and I went to see Mr Breast Consultant for the final outcome of all the further tests. It turns out that nothing out of the ordinary showed up on the pancreas MRI or thyroid ultrasound. The shadows in my pancreas and thyroid were nothing more than, well, just innocent shadows. No cancer there thankfully.

I've been checked from head to toe for cancerous tumours, but none have been found. Not even with the incredibly sensitive holy grail of all scans: the CT PET. Thus, given the combination of the markings on the cancer cells that were extracted from my lymph nodes, the location of the swollen lymph nodes, and a process of elimination, the cancer that I have is most likely, in all likeliness, probably, most certainly breast cancer.

Of course, there were questions about how I could possibly have breast cancer without them finding a tumour in one of my breasts (or anywhere else for that matter) and none of the other accompanying signs of breast cancer that a breast usually betrays: swelling, dimpling, puckering, redness, itching, soreness, inverted nipples, discharge or protruding veins.

In fact, I found my voice at this latest appointment.

"But surely it would have to be absolutely miniscule given that the CT PET scan didn't pick it up?" I asked confused. "Is it possible that my body has broken down the tumour itself?"

I secretly hoped that maybe my body was on my side and had gone to war with the tumour before it had been found. Mr Breast Consultant didn't think so.

Apparently, despite this being a very unusual situation, it is actually possible for this to happen. Some people have big tumours, some have medium ones, some have small ones and, it turns out that, in very few cases, some people don't have a noticeable tumour at all. Mr Breast Consultant said that in all likelihood, there was an incredibly small tumour in the left breast because the cancer cells were found in the left armpit lymph nodes.

Cancer cells can spread to the lymph nodes from miniscule tumours; they don't just spread from large tumours, which means that the severity of cancer is not just a matter of the size of the tumour. A large tumour may be caught before spreading to the lymph nodes and equally a tiny tumour may not be found until after it has spread to the lymph nodes.

I'm coming to understand that cancer is far more complex than I had originally thought. There are so many different permutations when it comes to symptoms, size, location and spread.

My husband asked about the stage and grade of the cancer. He (unlike me) had done a little bit of reading up on breast cancer before this appointment, and had come across these terms as being ones to describe the size and spread of the cancer. With his analytical mind, he too wanted to know exactly what we were dealing with. But no, with a fairly significant piece of the jigsaw puzzle missing, Mr Breast Consultant couldn't (wouldn't?) tell us the stage or grade and he didn't want to speculate without the full facts.

To be honest, I was a little relieved by that because talking about stages and grades just seemed to be a way of assessing the seriousness of the cancer, and in truth, I wasn't quite prepared for that conversation. Just like I wasn't ready to Google or research anything to do with breast cancer generally, or my specific situation. Yes, I know it goes against all normal Sara-is-good-at-a-life-project practice, but my head was swimming and I was still at the tell-me-what-I-need-to-know stage.

Whatever the explanation for the missing tumour, the crux of the matter is that I'm now officially a breast cancer patient. Which is, perhaps, ironic, given that I've now found out that this month is actually Breast Cancer Awareness Month.

One of my friends said, upon hearing this news, "Who'd have thought that we'd ever celebrate someone having breast cancer?"

But in a way, we did celebrate. It is such an almighty relief to now have a diagnosis. No more waiting to have a scan and then waiting for the results. The wait for test results is agonising, so having an official diagnosis from which we can move forward is very much a positive step.

"Breast cancer treatment is so advanced. It's one of the most treatable cancers, so if you're going to get cancer then this is the one to get."

I stared at my friend not knowing how to feel. I knew she meant well and was trying to make me feel better; perhaps she intended to make the whole thing sound less scary for both of us? In fact, if the shoe were on the other foot, I expect I would say something similar. After all, it must be incredibly difficult to know what to say to someone who has just been diagnosed with cancer. But *all* cancers are horrific, and I would rather not have any cancer at all.

At Wednesday's appointment, after discussing the missing tumour with Mr Breast Consultant, we moved on to the treatment plan. That was the conversation that I desperately wanted to have. He'd clearly given my situation some consideration and had discussed it with an oncologist. He had taken my case to his monthly breast consultant committee meeting, which is basically a regular meeting of regional breast consultants who gather to discuss cases, treatment developments and the world of breast cancer generally.

I liked the fact that he'd discussed my case with his breast consultant colleagues. I felt like I'd had a second, third, fourth opinion. Despite the absence of a tumour, Mr Breast Consultant had come up with a comprehensive treatment plan for me. He warned that it was going to be a tough ride, starting with surgery to remove the cancer-laden lymph nodes, followed by chemotherapy, then radiotherapy and some other treatments.

"So, do you think you'll be able to treat this then?" I'd asked at that appointment, hope gleaming in my eyes.

The extent of my cancer awareness was that cancer kills people—I mean, it's the biggest killer in the world. Even with my limited knowledge I was well aware that in treating cancer there were no guarantees, but rather a lot of unknowns. I knew there was no miracle cure for cancer and it couldn't be entirely prevented.

"Well, we're going to throw the book of treatment at you I'm afraid, but I'm confident that we can remove all the cancer from you. We aim to cure, not treat, this type of cancer."

And there it was. The answer that I'd been looking for all along.

He explained that the aim of the treatment he planned to give me wouldn't just remove all the cancer from me, but it would also help prevent any future spread or recurrence. There was no guarantee of no recurrence or spread, but he had given a good prognosis.

If I could park the recurrence/spread issue for the time being and focus on the getting-all-the-cancer-out-of-me part, then that was good enough for me. It was an answer that I could wedge into my heart and bring out when needed. Thank you, Mr Breast Consultant!

Following on from the official diagnosis of breast cancer at Wednesday's appointment, I realised that we couldn't keep the cancer secret any longer. We were going to have to break the news to people which I knew was going to be difficult. "I have breast cancer," are four words with which my brain seriously struggles. It's not something I ever thought that I would say.

Then there was the question of who to tell? Should I stand on the roof with a tannoy and make a big announcement? Or should I tell just close friends and family? What about work? My colleagues and my manager? School? Parents of my children's friends? How should we tell people? If I couldn't make the words come out of my mouth, should I use text and email? How would I word a text or email? Should I talk to people face to face or on the phone? How would they react? What would I have to deal with once the words had made it either out of my mouth or out via my thumbs? Would they treat me differently? Would I need to be strong and console them? Because I was feeling far from strong.

Worst of all, I couldn't bear to think about how and what we would say to the children. My two young, innocent children who had no idea that their world was about to be turned upside down.

After some careful deliberation following Wednesday's appointment, my husband and I decided that there wouldn't be any big announcement to the world, but, equally, we're not going to keep it a secret.

We drew up a list of people to tell:

1. The children (oh my, where do we start with this?).
2. My close friends who may be able to provide help and support.
3. My close family who need to know what is going on and will probably help as much as they can.
4. My work manager and colleagues so that they know why I will need a fairly significant amount of time off in the coming months.
5. Parents at school. I might need to rely on them for things like the school run.
6. The children's teachers so that they can keep an eye on the children.

I can't pretend that I don't have cancer. It is what it is. I want people to know so I don't have any awkward moments—I don't want to bump into someone and have to explain my situation. I want parents to know why I may not be able to invite their children to my house for play dates. I want friends to know why I may not be as chatty or sociable as usual and why I might not be up for coffee, dinner, and fun nights out quite so much. I want teachers to know why my children might not hand in their homework or learn their spellings on time. I want my colleagues to know that I'm not slacking. But we won't tell anyone tonight. Tonight is Bonfire Night. It's a night for wellies, scarves, warm jumpers, oohs and ahhs, hot chocolate with marshmallows, cold noses and fireworks.

CHECKLIST FOR FRIENDS AND FAMILY

What to say when someone has been diagnosed with breast cancer

- I am so sorry to hear this news.
- What an awful shock for you.
- Is there anything that I can do for you?
- *Tell* me what I can do for you.
- Can I take you to the hospital for any of your appointments/look after your children while you are at hospital/walk your dog for you?
- I'm here for you now, and I'll be here for you during your treatment.
- Would you like some company? Shall I pop in for a visit?
- I honestly don't know what to say.
- Do you want to talk about it?
- I'm thinking about you.

CHECKLIST FOR FRIENDS AND FAMILY

What NOT to say when someone has been diagnosed with breast cancer

- My aunt/mum/neighbour had breast cancer and she died.
- Breast cancer is a good cancer to get.
- Don't worry, I'm sure it will all be alright.
- It could be worse, at least. . .
- If you eat (insert one of a number of possible options here from 'turmeric' to 'an entirely vegan diet') it will cure your cancer.
- You'll beat this/I know you can fight this (anything involving 'battle language' isn't that great to hear).
- I know how you feel (only say this if you've been through it yourself).

CHAPTER 6

AT A BIT OF A LOOSE END

"A journey of a thousand miles begins with a single step."
Lao Tzu

It's a cold and wet Monday morning in November. Not one of those crisp autumnal mornings with a bright, blue sky showing off the colours of the orange and brown leaves. No, today is damp, misty and grey. The kind of day for staying inside and drinking hot tea with the radio for company.

The garden furniture is still in the garden. It hasn't been put away yet despite there being no hope of that last spell of sunshine. The grass is covered with more apples and more leaves. If they don't get raked up soon, they'll go mulchy and muddy. The trees look bare and forlorn, much like how I often feel at the moment. The children are at school. My husband is at work. I'm on my own at home and at a bit of a loose end.

I'm never at home on a Monday morning on my own. I'm usually at work, or if not in the office, I would be working from home, logged in on my laptop, talking to colleagues over email and via video link. But today I'm not working because Victor, my manager and a friend of fifteen years, gave me some fairly strict instructions the day after my initial diagnosis when I called him with The News.

"Absolutely no need to think about work under any circumstances. Don't even contemplate switching on your laptop or Blackberry. We have it covered. We'll cope."

I called him the day after D-Day because I knew that I would be needing a significant amount of time off work for all the tests and scans that Mr Breast Consultant had lined up for me. Victor kindly suggested that I take a bit of time off for the duration of those scans and to allow myself some time to absorb the diagnosis.

It was the right thing to do—with all the trips to hospital, I haven't known whether I'm coming or going for the past few weeks and I suspect that I would have been a bit of a liability at work. Given that the lymph node surgery is later this week (Mr Breast Consultant was keen to get me in for that as soon as possible), I won't be able to return to work for another few weeks, so a couple of days ago I did a handover of my workload for the immediate future.

So, here I am, on my own and at a bit of a loose end. Well, not quite on my own because I have my new sidekick, Breast Cancer, with me. Perched on my shoulder, where she's been since that Wednesday appointment with Mr Breast Consultant. She follows me everywhere, whispering scary things in my ear, clutching my heart, shaking me by the shoulders, sitting on my chest, distracting me every minute of the day, and waking me up at night.

Breast Cancer has a friend: dark, mean, over-bearing Fear. Fear of dying. Fear of leaving my husband. Fear of leaving my children without a mother. Fear of leaving before I'm ready or have fulfilled my hopes and dreams. Because despite Mr Breast Consultant telling me that he planned to 'cure' my cancer, I can't help but worry. I mean, it's freaking C-A-N-C-E-R and there are a whole host of what-if worries that accompany those six letters.

Worries ranging from things that deep down I know are irrational, like what if the whole missing breast tumour is just one big fat mistake and it's just been missed, to what if the treatment doesn't work? Then there's the what-if worry that I know I'll struggle with (despite my determination to park it for the time being); what if the cancer comes back or spreads?

I say that I'm at a bit of a loose end but that isn't strictly true either. There's plenty to do. The usual washing, tidying, cleaning, sorting, putting away and organising. In fact, there's more than usual to work through. Given the whirlwind of the past few weeks since my diagnosis, home life has been rather neglected.

It's impossible to focus on the mundanity of life with the diagnosis of cancer hanging around your neck. Washing has piled up, the house is a mess, the fridge is empty and dust covers every surface in sight.

I have my hands full today. I have a list, of course. A lovely, crisp, neat to-do list of normal daily chores and errands that I must achieve today and I think I can do it. I think that, today, I can get back that elusive friend of mine: Control. Control over our regular home life.

I'm also keen to get back control over what is happening to me and how this is going to impact our family life over the coming months. I have cancer, but I also have a treatment plan, so I'm going to focus on that. If I can take control of the treatment plan, then maybe I won't feel so terrified of what to expect from it, so I'm drawing up another list. A special 'get prepared for surgery this week' list.

It looks something like this:

1. Buy a folder for all my hospital paperwork. I'm going to need a big one. I haven't even started treatment and already I have forms and information sheets from the breast clinic and copies of letters to the GP. A folder with file dividers keeping everything in its place will make me feel better. I might even splash out and buy a new pen and notebook too.

2. Make space on the bookshelf for the Project Cancer Notebook, plus all my breast cancer paperwork and information so that it's kept in a safe, yet easily accessible, place. Amber, the very nice breast care nurse, gave me a folder about breast cancer. A very smart, colourful folder with a ring binder and lots of glossy information sheets neatly clipped inside. I haven't actually looked at anything in it. Contrary to the manner in which I usually approach life projects, I still haven't read anything about breast cancer yet; my shocked and overwhelmed brain remains not quite ready for that. I'll get there, but at the moment I've put my trust in Mr Breast Consultant and his colleagues to tell me what needs to be done in order to sort out this cancer situation of mine.

3. Buy one of those calendars with columns for each member of the family: me, my husband and one each

for the children. We need to have one place where we can see what everyone has going on each week so that if/when I'm not feeling well, my husband and Mum (when she comes over to help out) can make sure everyone is in the right place at the right time. Plus, my life will be overtaken with hospital appointments so I'll need to keep track of them.

4. Prepare an area in the kitchen where we can keep the calendar and constantly growing family admin documents. We need somewhere for all the school letters, birthday party invitations, bills, the children's activity letters and school timetables. We're going to need a 'family command centre.'

5. Prepare the spare room. Mum is coming to stay later this week when I go into hospital for my surgery. My mum is actually a real-life angel—the most wonderfully caring and loving human being on the planet. Her only mission in life seems to be to help my sister, me, our husbands and our children. She has been by my side since we sat facing Mr Breast Consultant when he told us that my lymph nodes were full of cancer cells. Her back has remained straight and her chin has been consistently held high. I need my mum right now and yet I feel horribly guilty for putting her through all this worry and stress.

6. Prepare to go into hospital for surgery to remove my cancer-laden lymph nodes. I've done a little bit of research about what I'll need to take to hospital when I go in for the surgery. I need an under-arm pillow, more pillows for the bed and some pyjamas that I can get on and

off after surgery, whilst my arm is out of action. I've already bought myself some new comfy clothes: soft, elasticated, stretchy, easy-wear trousers and warm, soft, woolly jumpers. I think illness inspires a need for the comfort of slouchy clothes in which you can mooch around the house. Stretchy trousers that aid sofa-lounging rather than skinny jeans which restrict all movement other than standing completely upright. I'll also need slippers. I expect to be at home for a certain proportion of the winter so slippers will be nice.

7. Buy teddies for the children. Yes, the children. Where do I start? Being diagnosed with cancer is obviously awful. I imagine that everyone who is diagnosed with cancer has the same fear of dying prematurely. That the treatment won't work and that their time is up/ that it will come back/that it will spread. That fear is so immense and vast and all-consuming. It's a black cloud hovering over us twenty-four hours a day but that fear is a fear for ourselves. It's a fear that *I* won't get through this and *I* will miss out on all *my* future hopes and dreams. Add children into the mix and the fear multiplies by an infinite amount because the fear is no longer just about our own personal situation and our own future, but it's about our children—their lives now and in the future. I wonder how my children, at their vulnerable, impressionable ages of nine and eleven, will take the news that their mother has cancer? How will they cope with the inevitable fear of losing their mother? How will my treatment disrupt their lives and how will they cope with that? How will the experience

affect them as they grow up? God forbid, how will they cope if I don't get through this?

So yesterday, my husband and I sat the children down and told them that I had a little lump of cancer cells in my armpit. We explained that the doctor would be taking them out and then I would be having some special medicine that would make me poorly, but at the end of all the treatment I would be better and back to normal.

Disney films and kids' TV programmes have a lot to answer for. Most children are only exposed to cancer through these mediums, where it is not unusual for mothers get cancer, go bald and die, and the story is all about life without the mother. So, the natural reaction of my children to the news of my cancer was immediate panic accompanied by, "Are you going to go bald and die?"

We told them that I wasn't going to die (because as things stand, Mr Breast Consultant is confident that this current cancer incident is not going to kill me) but that I was going to most likely go bald, and it would be the medicine rather than the cancer that would make me lose my hair. Children are brilliant. Amazing. Great. Once they had the reassurance that I probably wasn't going to die they focused on the bald issue, hesitantly asking questions and cautiously giving instructions.

"Will you have a wig?"

"Will you wear a hat?"

"Could you please not come to school—or anywhere—without a wig or hat? But the hat mustn't make you look bald underneath."

Nobody can see me bald. Phew. If their main concern is

being seen out with a bald mother, I think I can cope with that. So, the plan is to buy them a special teddy who will be their go-to for cuddles and chats when I am in hospital or not able to cuddle them while I'm having my treatment.

Where was I on my list?

8. Make room in the freezer for all the lovely meal deliveries that keep arriving at our door. Fairly soon after my diagnosis, my wonderful friend Antonia arrived on the doorstep with a casserole in one hand and banana muffins in the other. That was just the start of what has been the most overwhelming practical response to my situation: friends bringing me meals that I can pop in the freezer to bring out and reheat while I'm out of action after the surgery. Today I'm seeing a couple of close friends who've told me that they have some casseroles for our freezer to help with the aftermath of the surgery later this week. Whilst these particular friends have known about my cancer from the start of the scans and tests, we've now told a few more people on our need-to-know list so now the breast cancer cat is out of the bag.

As I expected, telling people that I have breast cancer has been weird. Every time I tell someone, it reiterates that this is really happening: that it isn't a dream. Because cancer is such a freaking big deal, from the moment I break the news, I become different to them. I'm no longer just Sara. I become Sara-With-Breast-Cancer. I don't want to be Sara-With-Breast-Cancer. I just want to be Sara. Or better yet, Sara-Without-Breast-Cancer.

Nonetheless, it's a relief to have told a few people. Some were fabulous and immediately knew exactly what to say to make me feel better. On the other hand, I now know that I'm not strong enough to deal with those who don't know how to react or can't hide their emotions. I've left my husband with the job of telling most people and hopefully the news will gradually filter out.

For now, my life is all about cancer. I can't change the fact that this is happening to me, but I've decided that I can control how I deal with it. My pause button has certainly been pressed. I have taken some deep breaths and tried to get my head around it. I feel better already just from writing out my to-do list. It's strange how the simple act of creating a list of things that I need to do can bring some calming control to the situation.

Despite having Breast Cancer and Fear perched on my shoulders, with all this organising I've taken the first step towards getting through this and there, at the back of my mind, is a little, wavering glimmer of hope that I might well be able to deal with this and come out the other side.

CHECKLIST

Shopping For Surgery

- Toiletries for your wash bag.
- Things to do at hospital, for example magazines, books, puzzle books etc.
- For node clearance and mastectomies: one or two bags to carry your drains, depending on whether you are having surgery on one or both sides.
- For mastectomies: a mastectomy pillow.

CHECKLIST

Things To Gather Together At Home, Or To Buy

- Small, soft, squidgy cushion or pillow that you can put under your arm after node clearance surgery.
- Flannels or sponges.
- Comfy clothes for convalescing at home.
- Extra pillows to help night-time sleeping.

CHECKLIST

Things To Organise

- Plan how you will sleep at night when you get home from hospital.
- Contact numbers for who to call about any questions to do with the recovery and drain.
- Plan and freeze some meals and do a grocery shop.
- Plan childcare.
- Clothing to accommodate the tubes and drain coming out of your armpit/chest.
- Check if the hospital will be providing compression socks.
- Ask someone to take you and bring you home from hospital.

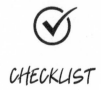

CHECKLIST

Hospital Bag

- Wash bag of toiletries (toothbrush, toothpaste, regular facial toiletries or face wipes, soap).
- Clean undies.
- Nightwear—ideally top and bottoms with the top being easy to open from the front.
- Dressing gown and slippers because you will probably have to walk to the operating theatre (not flip flops because you'll probably be wearing surgical stockings).
- Something to do like a book, magazine or downloaded film on an iPad/phone.
- Phone and charger.
- Snacks.
- Drinks.
- Notepad and pen for jotting down instructions and information from the nurses.
- Towel.
- Post-mastectomy bra.
- A small cushion that you can use in the car on the way home between the seatbelt and your chest.
- Something easy to wear when you leave hospital—ideally

something that buttons or zips up at the front, such as a skirt or jogging bottoms/baggies and flat, easy-to-slip-on shoes or boots.

- Small pillows for under your arms.
- Bags for the drains.
- Details of your prescription medication to give to the nurses.

A lot of these items can be bought online. There are too many places to list here, so check out www.tickingoffbreastcancer.com for a full list of online places to get some of these items (for example the drain bags, mastectomy pillows, post-mastectomy bras and post-surgery clothing).

CHAPTER 7

FINGERS CROSSED AND HOPING FOR THE BEST

"She stood in the storm, and when the wind did not blow her way – and it surely has not – she adjusted her sails."
Elizabeth Edwards

I'm in desperate need of a proper shower. A long, lush, stand-under-the-hot-water-for-twenty-minutes shower. The type of shower where you let the burning hot water fall down on you with your eyes closed, standing completely still, cleansing the whole world off your body, all the stress out of your muscles and the tiredness out of your bones.

I need to wash my hair. My hair requires a lot of work: it needs to be regularly washed, conditioned, prepped, pruned, tamed, straightened, oiled, sprayed and styled. I'm not one of those wash-and-go types. My hair is not easy to deal with but I've recently grown fond of it thanks to finally working out how to blow-dry it whilst straightening it at the same time. I used to despise and despair of it. I had short, mousey-brown ringlet curls when I was a child and I desperately wanted long, very straight, dark-brown hair. I was so desperate that when I was very little I used to attach a long, dark-brown towel to my head with a loop of elastic so that I could imagine it was my hair.

The ringlet curls grew into long frizzy curls when I was a teenager. I had the big Eighties-style curls, without the requisite Eighties perm. It was frizzy, untameable, out-of-control curly. I tried every type of product on the market from mousse to gel to oil to wax. None of them seemed to control the curls, or as I had hoped, to loosen the curls. My hair had a life of its own.

Over the years I went from long to shoulder-length to bob (not good for curly hair) back to long with a few more ups and downs along the way, but I like my brownish-blond, wavy, shoulder-length hair now. I'm desperately worried because, as far as I know, chemotherapy means losing my hair.

My last shower was Monday; today is Saturday. Having a wash in a bath with two inches of water every day just isn't the same. Especially when you need your mum there to help you navigate getting into and out of the bath (because you have a drain bag attached to your left armpit), and to scrub your back because only having one working arm means you can't reach around without getting the dressings wet. I have given up the pretence of maintaining dignity throughout this experience. Dignity was pushed out of the way when Breast Cancer and Fear stepped up onto my shoulders.

I can't believe that it was only a few weeks ago that Breast Cancer was finally named as the guilty culprit and hopped up onto my shoulder to keep me company. Things have moved quickly, which just adds to the air of surrealism that this experience continues to provide. Six days ago I had surgery to remove all the lymph nodes from my left armpit or, to use the correct term, an 'auxiliary node clearance.' Into the hospital I went, out came the nodes, in went a drain bag and out of the hospital I came a couple of days later.

The surgery was a fairly big deal for me (although obviously not as big a deal as those ladies undergoing a mastectomy). I'm a natural worrier so I was worried about:

1. The anaesthetic.
2. Having my body cut open.
3. How I would feel when I woke up.

Nevertheless, with my carefully packed overnight bag, I arrived at the hospital early in the morning so that Mr Breast Consultant could do his pre-op check of me on his early morning rounds.

After lots of waiting around—made all the more difficult because of the no eating or drinking rule when having a general anaesthetic—I had to change into the familiar hospital gown. This time I was given some delightful paper pants to wear. You know the ones: entirely see-through and you can't tell which is the back and which is the front. I was also given some dark emerald knee-high surgical stockings—the purpose of which was to prevent blood clots.

I'd brought my own dressing gown and slippers which I wore as I walked to the operating theatre. Yes, I actually walked to the operating theatre! I wasn't wheeled on a bed, or pushed in a wheelchair. This surprised me. I suppose because of all the medical dramas I've watched on TV over the years but it did make perfect practical sense.

I remember lying on the table in the little room next to the operating theatre, where I was being prepped for surgery by the anaesthetists. Just like in all the other previously un-experienced situations in which I had recently found myself, I was nervous because it was all so unfamiliar and I didn't know what to expect, but the two anaesthetists couldn't have been a better team.

The junior male anaesthetist held my hand and spoke soothing, comforting words to ease my nerves whilst the other, a formidable woman, discussed female equality in the workplace and the difficulties faced by working women and mothers. Fabulous. I could have quite happily lay there having that conversation rather than being wheeled in to theatre.

Waking up after surgery in the recovery room was weird. I felt like I'd just closed my eyes for a few minutes, not a matter of hours. I also felt numb, cold and very talkative. I babbled on at the nurse who was checking me over and then, this time it was like in the TV dramas, I was wheeled back to my bed and hooked up to a heart monitor, oxygen monitor and IV drip of pain medication.

I had some sort of strange contraption laid over my legs to prevent blood clots forming. It was dark outside by this time and I tried a cup of tea and sandwich but all I wanted to do was sleep. So I slept. But you don't get much sleep in hospital because the machines beep and the nurses regularly come and check your heart, oxygen levels and blood pressure.

At one point in the very early hours of the morning they wanted me to try going to the toilet. That was a real faff: unhooking the machines, wheeling the IV drip and stumbling on legs that felt like they hadn't been walked on in years rather than just a day. Life in my new, strange, cancer-reality was made even more odd when I checked my phone and saw the early results of the US presidential election: Trump had won. I thought I was dreaming. I went back to sleep.

I'd entered the hospital with a full house of lymph nodes. Then, after a couple of rather difficult days, I left hospital with a tube attached to my armpit and a bag into which the lost lymph fluid could flow, or rather drip.

Despite having been home now for a few days, I'm still attached to the bag. It's a bit like an IV bag, except it's attached to my armpit and the liquid within is bright orange, like Fanta but not fizzy. I can't feel where the tube goes into my armpit because most of my upper arm, armpit and shoulder are completely numb.

Using the Project Cancer Notebook, I make a daily note of how much Fanta drips into the drain bag to report back to Mr Breast Consultant. Once the amount consistently reaches a certain point—which I think indicates that lymph production is stabilising in this arm—Mr Breast Consultant will remove the drain and I will be drain-free.

I can't lift my arm further than halfway, although I have daily exercises to do which will help me to regain full arm movement.

All in all, there are all sorts of complications for getting dressed, washing, hugging, sleeping and generally getting by. However, the good news is that the little collection of evil cancer cells that had collected in my lymph nodes are no longer in me. Given the fact that they were the only evil cancer cells that could be located, Mr Breast Consultant tells me that he is confident that all the cancer has been removed.

Although I now know it's possible to have breast cancer without an apparent breast lump, it still feels a bit weird not to have had anything done to a breast so far—only surgery to remove my lymph nodes. I didn't have a mastectomy or a lumpectomy. There was nothing to remove with one of those procedures: they couldn't take out a breast lump if they couldn't find it and I know they looked very closely for it. I have the claustrophobic memories to prove it.

This does worry me a bit. Mr Breast Consultant suggested that they may not have found a tumour because it may be miniscule. Miniscule tumours are still tumours and, surely, they can grow into not-so-miniscule tumours? But Mr Breast Consultant told me that the discussion at the 'breast cancer consultant committee meeting' had resulted in a majority voting against a preventative mastectomy because without the evidence of any cancerous tissue, the combination of chemotherapy and radiotherapy would be sufficient preventative measures.

This means that I didn't have to endure the physical and emotional trauma of losing a breast plus all the pain and discomfort associated with that. I cannot begin to comprehend how it feels to lose a part of your body, especially a part that goes so far in defining who we are, whilst also dealing with the shock and trauma of a cancer diagnosis.

Given the lack of mastectomy or lumpectomy, I'm not sure to which Breast Cancer Club I belong. Maybe it's a small Breast Cancer Club of its own? One in which there are very few members and about which not much is known.

Mr Breast Consultant told me that he had come across this situation 'perhaps half a dozen times' in his career. Considering he is completely white-haired and wears a hearing aid, I'm inclined to think that his career may be as long as I am old, which means there aren't many cases like mine.

I'd very much like to feel special, but in fact all I feel is worried and scared. At least when they find a breast lump, they can take it out, test it, test the surrounding tissue, work out a plan of action, measure recovery and monitor recurrence. They have an algorithm for working out the chances of recurrence using the grade and stage of the cancer tumour. They can't even do that for me. With my mysterious cancer origination, I wonder whether there's an element of fingers crossed and hoping for the best on the part of everyone involved (me in particular).

Despite the mystery surrounding the origination of my cancer, it's still scary breast cancer. Going forward after surgery, I still have to endure a stack of what sounds like terrifying breast cancer treatment.

There has now been talk of meeting my oncologist, who will be monitoring my treatment from now on. 'My oncologist.' Now there's a phrase that I never expected nor wanted to say. Without offending all oncologists, I've really never wanted to meet one, let alone have one allocated to me.

Ten days ago, we started to spread the C-word. Within those ten days I have seen the most amazing side of human nature. Friends have visited. I've had cards, texts, emails, letters, flowers, gifts and food delivered to the doorstep. Friends and family have written the kindest, most caring words to me. They've sent the most thoughtful cards and chosen the most loving gifts.

I've been completely overwhelmed by the reactions of my friends and family. Love and Support have most certainly arrived on the doorstep with their arms wide open, ready to wrap us in their warm embrace. The abrupt deviation off my life path and onto the cancer path has impacted these people. People who, like me, were running along the treadmill of life, taking their health and family for granted, have been stopped in their tracks by the shock that someone just like them, has been diagnosed with the big C. They've stepped off the treadmill and out of their cosy bubbles to face the cancer (the it-could-have-been-any-one-of-us cancer) in their midst.

There has been a definite rallying around with plenty of offers of practical support, like the school-run rota—an absolute lifeline—offers to have the children during hospital appointments and I've had more offers to take me to hospital appointments than I can shake a stick at.

Food keeps arriving for the freezer and male friends have generously offered to take my husband out for a drink. I think it's a manly way of saying, "I'm here for you mate."

Telling people the news, receiving gifts and being the centre of attention—which I am really uncomfortable with —is all a bit too familiar. It's a bit like the to-do list for the most dreadful engagement ever:

1. A proposal—the diagnosis.
2. The fanfare of telling people.
3. The arrival of gifts and cards.
4. People make a big fuss.

Unfortunately, unlike an engagement, which leads to the fun of organising a wedding then celebrating the future life of the happy couple, I have the joy of organising the next ten months of my life whilst I recover from surgery and then undergo chemotherapy and radiotherapy, whilst questioning how long I have left of my future.

But you know what? With the loving support of my truly

wonderful family and friends, I'm going to dig really deep and find the strength to get through this. I know that, without a doubt, I have a caring support network on whom I'll be able to lean on. I know that my husband and children will be looked after whilst I go through whatever treatment has in store for me. I know that I'll be looked after.

Breast Cancer and Fear, you may have made yourselves comfortable on my shoulders, but let me tell you now, you have an awful lot of Love and Support to contend with.

CHECKLIST FOR FRIENDS AND FAMILY

Practical Ways To Help Someone With Cancer

Practical help really is the biggest gift you can give your friend or family member while they go through treatment for cancer; be it surgery, chemo or radiotherapy. Remember that when you offer help, make it clear that you genuinely mean it. Even after the tenth time they decline it; they might accept your eleventh offer. Ways in which you could offer practical help:

- Deliver meals they can freeze and reheat at a later date. Check if any she or her family have any food allergies or taste issues arising out of treatment.
- Help with childcare after school, at weekends and during school holidays.
- Offer to organise a rota with other friends to help out with childcare, school runs, children's club runs, chemo trips, radiotherapy trips, medical appointments. One of the kindest, most helpful things that three friends did for me was to arrange a school run rota and drive my children to and from school every day. I am eternally grateful for that.
- If she is fatigued and not able to get up and about very

much, offer to help in the home, such as putting on the washing, emptying the dishwasher, ironing and hoovering.

- Offer to pick up their groceries, toiletries, prescriptions and anything else, which saves them from making a trip to the shops.
- Offer to take them to any medical appointments and take notes.
- If you live close by, then you could offer to be a night-time emergency contact, so that if they need to go to hospital you can either be the person they contact to take them, or you can babysit their children in the middle of the night.
- Can you take their dog for a walk? Mow the grass? Help with any gardening jobs? Put their garden furniture away?

CHAPTER 8

THE STAR ON TOP OF THE CHRISTMAS TREE

"Anxiety happens when you think you have to figure everything out all at once. Breathe. You're strong. You got this.
Take it day by day."
Karen Salmansohn

We're getting the Christmas tree today. It's slightly earlier than we would usually get it but we're a few days into December so at least we're in the Christmas month. My husband has gone to pick one up from a local farm whilst the children and I unpack the decorations. Michael Bublé is keeping us company and the winter candle has been lit, sending its gorgeous cinnamon-citrus scent around the house.

This is a part of Christmas that I love: the planning, the decorations, the lights, the Christmas songs, the smells and anticipation. The part before the songs get annoying, the decorations start to make the house feel cluttered and dusty, the pine needles cover the floor, and before the whole thing just gets too much.

I love unwrapping each of the fragile tree decorations and reminding myself where some of the special decorations came from: my children's first Christmases, the decorations made by them and the ones given to us as gifts. Then there's that distinctive smell that wafts out of the box as we unpack the decorations: the musty cinnamon smell of Christmas.

The Fanta drain has gone. It was removed a couple of weeks ago. When Mr Breast Consultant removed the drain, I was worried that all the lymph in my arm would seep through the stitched-up incision where the tube had previously been snugly in place. Actually, I was slightly concerned that the lymph fluid would gush out.

The breast care nurse suggested that I pop a sanitary towel under my armpit to catch any seeping lymph. A big one, not a discrete one. Gina kindly popped to the chemist for me and bought three packs of the biggest, most brick-like sanitary towels she could find and I worked out how to stick them to the inside of my top. Good times. I was walking around with a sore, stiff, numb upper arm and a sanitary towel strategically placed in the armpit region.

After a few days, the seepage stopped and I started to get a swollen bulge in my armpit where lymph fluid had collected—presumably because the incision had healed to a point where no fluid could get past and escape. The bulge grew to be the size of a grapefruit! No wonder I needed a small pillow to put under my arm.

I've since been back and forth to the breast clinic to have the seroma (as I now know the bulge to be called) aspirated. This is where Mr Breast Consultant inserts a needle into my armpit and sucks out the lymph fluid with a syringe (or two or three syringes in my case, due to the size of the seroma).

I've been feeling rather smugly brave about having the

aspiration done. Although it's a pretty big needle, my entire upper arm is still completely numb so luckily I haven't been able to feel a thing whilst he carries out the procedure. In fact, I have occasionally watched, with fascination, as he draws out the gross gunk into the syringe.

One of the surprising side effects of the lymph node surgery has been the difficulty I've had in moving my arm. Immediately following surgery and for a few weeks thereafter, my arm felt as if it had completely lost the ability to rise up in the air and above my head. Forcing my arm up further and further against its will was like trying to bend a finger backwards. This stiffness was caused by something called cording.

After lymph node removal surgery, you can see and feel long, tight cords in your arm (which actually feel, and look, like guitar string cords under the skin). They are so tight that they significantly limit the movement of that arm. I had to undergo physiotherapy for this.

I saw the lovely Gill for physio. With her soft, lilting northern accent, she would give me a running commentary as she gently squeezed and pulled these cords in the hope of snapping them, whilst I lay on the treatment table. When a cord snapped, we would hear a gentle pop. Gill felt very satisfied by these pops and each one gave her the incentive to move on and snap more. I just felt like I wanted to vomit.

Gill instructed me to do exercises at home to help with the cording. The fear of forever having restricted arm movement has kept me practising these monotonous exercises day in, day out. She told me the best thing I could do was to use my arm. She suggested that I take a cloth and clean the windows round and round, moving my arm up as far as it would go, every day. As one to follow instructions, that's what I've been doing.

The other thing about having no lymph nodes in one of my arms is that I'm apparently now at risk of something called lymphoedema. Mr Breast Consultant spoke to me about this just before I went in for surgery and I have to admit, I didn't take it all in. I have, however, looked it up since and read the leaflet he gave me.

Lymphoedema is a collection of fluid in the soft tissue of the arm or breast after the lymph vessels in the arm have been cut and the lymph nodes have been taken out. It's a risk for life: lymphoedema swelling can occur at any time after surgery and once it happens, you'll always have the swelling. There are lists of things to do, and not to do, to help reduce your risk of developing lymphoedema, and if it does develop it can be controlled with compression garments—essentially a very tight arm sleeve.

Today, as I unpack the Christmas decorations—with an arm that is, I'm pleased to say, moving very well thank you—I am joined by Breast Cancer and Fear. I'm trying not to pay them any attention. I want to enjoy today's decorating ritual. Breast Cancer and Fear are unwelcome and I'm trying very hard to ignore their scary whispers that this may be the last time I unpack the decoration box.

Unfortunately, they've been keeping me company most of the time recently. Probably because the cancer diagnosis has now fully sunk in and my little what-if wobbles are a bit of a fixture at the moment. Breast Cancer and Fear have now brought Sadness along to the party too.

Sadness: that bleak, downcast, glum pal of theirs. I can't

listen to music; the lyrics to every song being played on the radio seem to be about people going away and leaving someone behind. I can't watch, read or listen to the news. It's all so sad and depressing.

I've been spending most of my time at home recently because of the limitations in my arm movements and the general crappiness of how I've been feeling. I'm rarely on my own at home though, which has been a great distraction from Breast Cancer, Fear and Sadness.

Although my husband has been back at work for the past month since the operation and the children are at school, I've had no end of visitors. Lovely friends coming to see me bringing plenty of love, support, lunch, cakes, biscuits (thank goodness for those elasticated waist band trousers) and generally keeping me company whilst I've been recovering from surgery.

In between the visitors, I have been planning for chemo and organising Christmas. Chemo starts in a week. I am petrified.

Up until two weeks ago (which was when we went to see Mr Oncologist for the first time), I knew nothing about chemotherapy. The extent of my chemotherapy knowledge came from TV and movies: chemo makes you bald and very sick. Yes, Mr Breast Consultant had mentioned the need for chemotherapy at the beginning of November, and you might expect that, being a bit of an expert at life projects, I would have immediately trawled through the Internet to find out as much as I could about chemotherapy. I didn't do that. I was feeling decidedly overwhelmed during the period of time after the diagnosis and throughout surgery. I wasn't able to think straight and I was struggling to get my head around the surreal situation. My head was in no position for me to start Googling chemotherapy.

However, when we got the date for my first appointment with the oncologist and I knew that I couldn't hide from chemotherapy any longer, I accepted that I should address it, so I made a list of questions to take with me. It went something like this:

1. How will the chemotherapy be given to me?
2. How long will the chemotherapy process last at each appointment?
3. How often will I have chemotherapy and for how many months?
4. Which chemotherapy drugs will I be given? Are there different drugs for different cancers?
5. What are the common side effects associated with my chemo drugs?
6. Will I feel terribly sick a lot of the time? Can I take any anti-sickness medication?
7. What do I do if I suffer from side effects?
8. Who should I get in touch with if I have side effects, and how?
9. How often, and in which department in the hospital, do I have blood tests?
10. What do they do blood tests for?
11. What time should I arrive on the morning of my chemo?
12. Is there anything in particular that I should bring with me when I come for chemo?
13. Will I be sitting in a room with other breast cancer patients, or a mix of patients?

14. How often will I see the oncologist?
15. Can I work during chemo?
16. Can I take any over-the-counter medication? For example, my asthma medication, hay fever medication, paracetamol, indigestion tablets and so on?
17. Finally, but very, very importantly, will my hair fall out? (I actually wanted to ask this question first, but I worried that it would look as if I had my priorities upside down if I asked this question before some of the others.)

We went to see Mr Oncologist a couple of weeks ago at the big cancer centre where I had my CT PET scan. I was more prepared for the cancer-ish-ness of the hospital on this visit. Mr Oncologist was very nice. He had a soothing voice: good for panic-stricken cancer patients. He was also as old as my dad so I took comfort in his years of experience and knowledge.

"A number of my female patients are concerned about losing their hair, and I'm afraid, Sara, that it's most likely that you will lose your hair." He came out with it fairly early on in the appointment. I didn't even have to ask the question. "But there are some wonderful, very realistic wigs available which look like real hair. In fact, I can't tell which ladies are wearing wigs from those who haven't lost their hair."

Losing hair. Wigs. Yet another example of how everything constantly feels so far removed from real life these days.

My husband had, of course, taken the Project Cancer Notebook to the oncologist appointment and throughout the appointment he took copious notes, as we asked all the questions on my list.

My husband is doing well in his role as project manager of Project Breast Cancer. As well as not being able to actually concentrate on anything at the moment, I'm finding it difficult to retain any information that's given to me. So, my husband is coming to all consultant appointments, writing everything down in the Project Cancer Notebook, typing up the notes into easily digestible emails for me and generally being my rock. He's upbeat and positive. He's carrying on life as normal. He's being strong. He's being brilliantly perfect.

At the meeting with Mr Oncologist we found out that there isn't just one type of breast cancer, nor is there a one-size-fits-all breast cancer treatment. There are, in fact, all sorts of different types of breast cancer with specific treatments for each type.

Half of me was surprised (yeah, I would have known this if I'd read my glossy breast cancer folder or gone on Google), and half of me wasn't surprised (off the back of finding out that there is an array of breast cancer symptoms, sizes, locations and spreads). I suppose I thought breast cancer was, well, breast cancer. Apparently not.

The cancer cells in the lymph nodes that were removed from me were tested by the pathology department of the hospital to ascertain the type of breast cancer I have. Amazingly, they can do that without testing the tumour. The type that I have requires me to have two types of chemo drugs, which will be given to me sequentially over the course of eighteen sessions over six months. Having chemotherapy is meant to be a preventative measure to mop up any stray cancer cells that may have spread further than the lymph nodes.

It turns out that breast cancer cells and tumours are sneaky, clever little buggers and have receptors, which are proteins in the breast cancer cells capable of picking up signals from certain chemicals in the body telling the cancer cells to grow. We don't want any of those particular chemicals in my body telling any stray cancer cells to grow.

My breast cancer tested positive for oestrogen receptors and HER2 receptors. To deal with the oestrogen-positive receptors, I will be taking a daily hormone therapy tablet called Tamoxifen for between five and ten years. Tamoxifen blocks the effects of oestrogen on these receptors, helping to stop oestrogen from encouraging any breast cancer cells to grow.

The HER2 receptors are on the breast cancer cell surface and they stimulate growth of a tumour. I will be getting a biotherapy injection called Herceptin every three weeks for one year, which works by attaching itself to the HER2 receptors, so that any stray cancer cells are no longer stimulated to grow.

Oh, and let's not forget the course of radiotherapy that will start within a month of finishing chemo.

So much information to take in and so much treatment to undergo over such a long period of time.

"Don't Google your type of breast cancer. If you do, then you'll find out-of-date information that calls it an aggressive cancer, which it isn't. There's very good treatment for it, but the treatment is relatively new," he instructed me firmly as he told me about the HER2-positive pathology results.

No problem. I wasn't keen to get to know Dr Google anyway, so I was happy to oblige.

My first chemo appointment is going to take place in one week's time on December 14th. Just in time for Christmas. A little early Christmas present, if you like.

In preparation for chemo, a few days ago, my husband and

I visited the chemotherapy ward at the hospital. The visit to the chemo ward and meeting the chemo nurses was—let's be honest—quite daunting. I was given a lot of information about the chemo drugs that they would be pumping into me. My shiny new breast cancer folder is getting pretty full.

They gave me a book with a traffic-light system for side effects: those in the green list are ones I will need to mention to the nurses on my subsequent visit, if I have amber ones I will need to call up the chemo nurses for advice, and if I have any red ones I will need to go to A&E. There are a lot of red ones. All of the side effects sound horrible, no matter the colour, and here I am voluntarily allowing someone to pump me full of the chemicals that are going to cause these side effects. For six months. Which is half a freaking year!

Looking at the information from the chemo ward visit and the traffic-light book, I'm expecting to not feel my best and to need some help, so Mum has offered to come and stay like she did after my surgery. The plan is for Mum to stay from the first day of chemo until we can cope without her. She's going to do it for every cycle. Every time I go into hospital to be pumped with chemicals; she'll move in for as many days as needed until we can cope. As I said, she is an angel.

The school-run rota that friends set up after surgery will carry on for as long and as often as I need the help. I don't think that my friends doing this rota realise what an absolute lifeline this is for us.

The new family calendar has proved very efficient and is now centre stage of the family command centre in the corner of the kitchen.

The freezer is full to the brim with delicious-looking

casseroles, lasagnes, pies and yummy dishes thanks to my wonderful friends.

We are logistically as ready to go as we possibly can be. I, on the other hand, don't feel quite so ready to go. I've now read all the practical advice I could find on the web about getting through chemo. I've made dozens of shopping lists and shopped for everything I need. I've packed a chemo bag to take to the hospital. I've bought lots of healthy snacks and I have cupboards of food recommended for ladies going through breast cancer chemotherapy. I have plenty of soft, comfy clothes and slippers for my convalescing days. I have bottles of antibacterial hand wash scattered throughout the house to ensure that not a single teeny tiny germ can survive here.

I even have a personalised relaxation recording downloaded onto my phone—a friend recorded it for me to help me cope with any stress or anxiety brought on by the chemo. I've added the telephone numbers of those I need to call in different side-effect situations to my phone and I've put a copy of the numbers in the family command centre. I have a bucket load of things to help me through my recovery days including magazines, books, DVDs, sweets, ice lollies made with homemade orange juice, a new subscription to Netflix and Amazon Prime, and even a bell to ring when I need a family member to come running with cups of tea and biscuits.

I must point out that I didn't buy the bell; a friend gave it to me because she thought that a bell would come in handy. I'll admit, I'm looking forward to giving it a go.

Yet, despite all this organising, I'm not ready to start chemo. I'm not ready to experience the nausea, the hair loss, the mouth ulcers, the aching joints, the fatigue, the horrible skin, my nails falling off, the headaches, the dry throat, or any of the other side effects listed in my traffic-light book. Despite all the practical preparations, I'm mentally unprepared for embarking upon it.

However, I suppose that the sooner I start the treatment, the sooner the treatment finishes. And the sooner I start, I'll know what to expect, how to get through the side effects and how long any side effects will last. I just have to remember that I don't need to figure everything out right now. I'm doing this. I just need to take a deep breath and remind myself that I *can*.

Right, back to organising Christmas. We've decided to have a quiet Christmas this year. Given the proximity of Christmas to chemo we are going to have just the four of us at home for Christmas Day. The four of us and our Christmas jumpers, huddled together inside, away from the harshness of winter and the beastliness of cancer. I'm really looking forward to it. I just need to get the little matter of my first chemo appointment out of the way.

Putting the Christmas tree and the decorations up today is almost the last thing we need to do. I have never been so organised for Christmas so early in December!

1. Presents bought and wrapped.
2. Food for Christmas Day lunch ordered, to be delivered.
3. Cards bought, written and posted.

I've been religiously doing my arm exercises every day since my operation. The movement in my arm is almost back to normal, so I'll have no problem popping the star on top of the tree today.

CHECKLIST FOR PLANNING CHEMOTHERAPY

Things To Gather At Home Or To Purchase

- Warm socks or slippers—you can get cold with some chemo drugs.
- Water bottle.
- Notebook and pen to make a note of any questions as and when you think of them.
- iPad/tablet/laptop with downloaded films and earphones to take to chemo.
- Warm scarf/shawl to keep you snug during chemo and whilst recovering at home.
- Blankets for the sofa—again to keep snug during your recovery days.
- Distractions for the rough days (TV box sets, films, books, magazines, etc).
- Antibacterial hand gels—small and large sizes—to have around the house or in your car, handbag, chemo bag etc.
- Gentle toothpaste and mouth wash—either for sensitive teeth or an organic brand.
- Soft toothbrush (possibly a child's brush) because chemo can make your gums soft and sore.

- Prescription medication so you don't run out when you least feel up to getting to the doctor and pharmacy.
- Tissues.
- Gentle shampoo and conditioner—your hair and scalp will be really sensitive.
- Eye drops for dry eyes.
- Gentle shower gel and moisturiser—chemo can make your skin sensitive.
- Decent thermometer. Shop around for this as you'll often find reductions in supermarkets. You'll need to keep an eye on your temperature if you feel unwell.
- Travel sickness wristbands. These can help with any nausea.
- Stock up on over-the-counter medication which has been approved by your oncologist so that you have it as and when needed: Indigestion/heartburn remedies, paracetamol, throat sweets and throat spray.
- Soft head caps and scarves to prepare for hair loss if you are not using the cold cap.
- PICC line covers (if you are having a PICC line). Make sure you have some day-wear ones and some waterproof ones for showers. For places to get these, there are links on www.tickingoffbreastcancer.com

CHECKLIST FOR PLANNING CHEMOTHERAPY

Things to Organise

- Go shopping for all the bits you need for your chemo bag and for at home during your chemo recovery days.
- See the dentist before chemo starts because you may be advised not to have any dental work done whilst having chemo.
- Sort out your freezer to make room for frozen meals.
- Make some meals to freeze for those days when you won't be up to cooking.
- Apply for your free NHS prescription certificate (in the UK).
- Plan childcare and help with the school run—don't be afraid to ask friends and family for help because they'll probably want to help.
- Organise a 'family command centre' at home so that other people can help with keeping track of family life if there are days when you just can't get up and about.
- Save important hospital contact numbers in your phone and keep a written note of them somewhere around the house.
- Prepare yourself for the possibility of needing to have

your head shaved when you start losing your hair by asking around at local hair salons, or asking a friend or family member to do it.

- Look into the option of getting a wig, if you want one, in case your hair falls out.
- Make some frozen fruit juice ice lollies and freeze some fresh pineapples. These can be soothing for a sore mouth.
- The hospital may give you a 'chemo card' that shows your personal information, the hospital contact details and the name of your chemo drugs. Make sure you have your chemo card on you at all times when you leave the house so that if you are in an accident or are taken ill, the paramedics know to take your chemo drugs into account when they treat you.
- Ask a friend or family member to take you and bring you home from chemo.
- If you are due to have chemo through the winter, ask your GP about getting flu jabs for your family members and possibly yourself (check with your oncologist first), because you don't want the flu during chemo.
- Pack your chemo bag:
    1. Snacks.
    2. Something nice to drink—such as herbal tea or cordial.
    3. Warm socks or slippers.
    4. Shawl or blanket.
    5. Hard-boiled sweets and mints to help with the aftertaste of chemo.
    6. Lip balm and hand cream.

7. Notebook and pen for notes about treatment.
8. Hospital chemotherapy book—the one the hospital gives you to record your appointments.
9. Antibacterial hand gel.
10. Magazine or a book.
11. Something to do like a crossword, puzzle book, a mindfulness colouring book and pencils, or an iPad/tablet/laptop with downloaded films and earphones.
12. Possibly something for lunch depending on how long you will be in hospital and whether or not you will be provided with lunch. Check with the chemo nurses before you go for your first round of chemo.
13. If you are planning to use the cold cap then you may need to take conditioner and a comb if the hospital doesn't provide them, plus a warm scarf/shawl. Check with the chemo nurses what you need to take.

- Pack your emergency hospital bag so it is ready in case of an emergency. You'll need to remember to also take your chemo records if you have to go to hospital:
  1. Nightwear.
  2. Wash bag.
  3. Book or something to do while waiting.
  4. Set of clean underwear and clothes.
  5. Antibacterial hand gel and antibacterial wipes.

CHAPTER 9
JUST THE ONE NEW YEAR'S RESOLUTION

"To lose confidence in one's body is to lose confidence in oneself."
Simone de Beauvoir

To-do list:

1. Back to school.
2. Tidy the garden (oh dear, still not done!).
3. Plan New Year's Resolutions.
4. Try cold cap.
5. Shave head.

The children went back to school today. The Christmas holidays are over. We're a week into the New Year and it's officially winter. It's been quite a mild winter. Personally, I like a harsh, cold winter: piercing blue skies and a low sun. I love snuggling up inside while winter covers everything outside. I adore being out and about, wrapped up from head to toe, breathing in the crisp air. I love the way the sun shines in winter and everything has a sharpness about it. I even like the foggy days when it seems as if the clouds have fallen from the sky onto the ground.

The garden has a rather desolate, neglected look about it today: the furniture is still sitting outside on the patio with no attempt having been made to put it away for winter. Nobody has raked the leaves or picked up the rotting apples scattered across the lawn. The trees in the garden are completely bare, forming dark silhouettes against the low sunlight.

I'm becoming quite mesmerised, staring out into the garden. I've taken to sitting in the kitchen quite a lot over the past few weeks, drinking tea and watching autumn disappear. In fact, I've taken to sitting down anywhere and everywhere recently. All my energy has been sucked out of me, as if someone turned on a tap one day and all the energy poured out. It's all I can do to move around the house slowly and gently from bed to sofa to chair, over and over again.

It's blissfully, comfortingly, strangely quiet today. The tornado of chemotherapy has well and truly torn through our home over the past few weeks, leaving in its wake four rather dazed people. Thankfully, going back to school today means that some sort of semi-normal routine can resume for the children and my husband.

I, on the other hand, am just getting used to my new, completely strange and rather unpleasant routine of chemotherapy cycles and side effects that promise to accompany me well into this year. I am two cycles into a total of six cycles of my first chemo drug.

A chemo cycle is the period of time from the day on which the chemo drugs are administered followed by a number of days while the chemo drugs do their thing. My current cycles are three weeks, which means that I have chemo on day one, then I wait twenty days for the drugs to work their way around my body doing their zapping and blasting and killing off any bad stuff, and then I do it all again.

So here we are, a New Year and a new me. No bland New Year's resolutions this year. No vacant promises to drink less alcohol, exercise more or take up a new hobby. I have only one resolution: to make it through this year of treatment and into the next, when hopefully I can put all this cancer crap behind me.

I don't recognise myself at the moment. I'm tired and slow. I'm puffy and exhausted. I'm aching and I'm scared and I'm bald. Other than a sprinkling of teeny, tiny, stubble patches here and there across my scalp, all my hair has gone.

Whilst I'm not happy about losing my hair, I think before I even started chemo I had almost accepted that I would lose it. It's strange, but at some point along the cancer path you are confronted with the fact that you will most likely lose your hair. All thoughts of dying and survival are pushed aside while the thought of your hair falling out takes up all your brain space.

One of the first questions that my children asked me when we broke the news was, "Will your hair fall out?"

One of the most critical questions on my list for Mr Oncologist was, "Will I lose my hair?"

The first question I asked my chemo nurses was, "When will my hair fall out?"

It's just hair. Losing hair is not forever, but dying and survival are, so why all the vain fuss about going bald? What is it about becoming bald that scares us cancer patients so badly? Is it the loss of our personal identity that baldness cruelly brings? Is it an association between the baldness and death? Is it because the baldness represents cancer? And we can no longer pretend that cancer isn't really happening? Is it because baldness tells the rest of the world that we are sick? Are we worried that losing our hair will change our personality? Do we feel defined by our looks so the loss of our hair changes who we are?

But there is a magic hat. A magic hat that you can wear during chemotherapy, which stops your hair from falling out. A magic, very cold hat which allows you to keep your hair. It's called the cold cap.

'Cold' just doesn't cut the mustard when talking about the cold cap. It's a mind-numbing cold. The whole point of the cold cap is to reduce the temperature of your scalp so less blood flows there, which in turn helps to prevent the chemotherapy drugs from reaching the hair follicles.

I loved my hair. I loved my brownish-blond, wavy, shoulder-length hair. I didn't want it to go, so, I tried the magic cold cap. It's like a long tube of car antifreeze which is wound round and round into the shape of a head, covered by a horse-riding hat. You have to wet your hair and slather it in conditioner before you put the hat on your head, and the nurse makes sure that there are no gaps between the tube of antifreeze and your head. Then the cap is switched on and the liquid in the tube gets very cold.

I sat for twenty minutes with what felt like a block of ice on my head, my neck barely able to stand the weight. My head was completely numb from the cold and throbbing with pain. I gave it twenty minutes. I gave my lovely, brownish-blond, wavy, shoulder-length hair twenty minutes. Then I gave a silent apology to my hair and I asked the nurses to take it off and that was it. Goodbye hair. (I ought to say here that whilst the cold cap was not for me, everyone feels the cold differently and many people cope with wearing a cold cap during all of their chemo sessions.)

When I asked the chemo nurse when I should expect my hair to start falling out, she told me in a matter-of-fact manner entirely at odds with my rising panic that in her experience of seeing it happen, it would most likely start to fall out around the eighteenth day after the first cycle of chemo.

Day seventeen after my first cycle of chemotherapy (New Year's Eve in fact) saw the first desolate strands of hair start falling out; a small handful attached itself to my fingers as I tried to pull it back into a ponytail that morning. It came out in clumps from that point on. Small handfuls. I couldn't touch my hair without it leaving my head and attaching itself to my hands. I couldn't run my fingers through my hair without it coming out. I couldn't wash it because every follicle holding every strand had become so fragile that the slightest nudge would release the delicate strands of hair out of my scalp. I certainly couldn't use a hair dryer or comb through any hair products. I was waking up in the mornings to strands on the pillow, and strands would cover my clothes at the end of the day.

What I wasn't warned about, or prepared for, was the excruciating scalp pain. It was a crazy, infuriating, itching pain all over my head from front to back and from side to side. But I couldn't do much about it because trying to relieve the itch meant losing more strands of hair.

Within a day or so of the first handfuls falling out and the start of the awful scalp pain, I, unhappily and reluctantly, decided that my hair had to go. I would get it shaved off rather than wait for it to fall out, bald patch by bald patch. Given the number of bald patches that had appeared here and there across my head, anything other than shaving was not really an option.

However, despite making this decision around January 1st or 2nd, I couldn't easily do anything about getting it shaved right then because:

1. I had decided that I was definitely going to a hair salon to have it shaved professionally. No friend or family member was coming close to me with a razor. But it was the weekend after New Year, and Monday was a bank holiday so everywhere was closed.

2. My next cycle of chemo was imminent. Tuesday would be 'bloods' at the hospital and chemo was due on the Wednesday, so I ruled out that week for a head shave, knowing I would be feeling grim from chemo and would rather sort out my hair when I was feeling relatively okay.

3. I hadn't done anything about getting a wig because of Christmas and the New Year. I had always been adamant that as soon as I'd had my head shaved, I would be wearing a wig all day, every day. I really didn't want to go and get my head shaved without having a wig to pop straight onto my bald head.

I crossed my fingers that I could hold out until mid-January when I would have got over the worst of the chemo and, by which time, I would have sorted out my wig. I hoped that my hair would just thin gradually and that the bald patches could be camouflaged to get me through to a time when I felt well enough to do something about it, and I could get organised.

You can be prepared for losing your hair. You can accept that you will lose it but actually, making the move to go and get it shaved off, now that's another matter. I suppose there's a tiny flicker of hope that the hair will stop falling out, that those bald patches appearing over your scalp can be covered and that you won't lose it all.

For me, that hope was cruelly dashed when I woke one morning—the day after my second cycle of chemo—to what can only be described as a bird's nest on my head. My hair didn't feel like hair. It had changed overnight to straw. Brittle, hard straw, which was stuck in a matted, messy mesh. I couldn't run one finger through it. My lovely brownish-blond, wavy, shoulder-length hair had completely transformed.

My mum and my sister, Emma, came to the rescue. Emma had obviously been terribly shocked by my diagnosis and we'd seen each other a few times after D-Day.

Emma came to see me the day after my second cycle of chemo to my welcome of, "What the bloody hell am I going to do about this bird's nest?" I mumbled this rather than shouted, from my foetal position on the bed, feeling truly awful from the chemo. I felt so sick that I could barely lift my head to register the bird's nest in the first place.

Between Mum and Emma, they managed to locate a local hair salon with someone who could shave my head that day.

Piling into the car with both children—it was unhelpfully still the school holidays—we popped to the hospital to get some stronger anti-sickness medication, plus the routine post-chemo injection in my tummy which helps my body make extra white blood cells to boost my immune system. Then we moved on to the hairdressers.

While Mum stayed in the car with the children—so they wouldn't be traumatised by the whole episode—Emma and I went into a little private room upstairs in the salon, away from the regular wash and blow dry clients. It only had one chair in front a mirror. Either side of the mirror were fitted shelves on which were, maybe, fifty polystyrene heads holding an assortment of wigs of all colours, lengths and styles.

Emma thought it would be a good opportunity for me to try a few on. I've only ever worn a wig once in my life. It was a synthetic deep gold, short, curly one in my early twenties for a Seventies disco night and I'd have gone up in flames had I stood near a naked flame.

We chose a few that we thought most closely resembled my old hair, or so we thought, but once they were on my head, I didn't look like me. I looked like a cross between a newsreader in a Nineties American TV programme and a seventy-year-old woman.

Putting the wigs back onto their polystyrene heads, we agreed it might be best to park the wig situation until I was feeling physically and mentally stronger.

I let Emma take one photo of me midway through the head shave. Some people hold shaving parties and film the whole thing, whilst others take loads of photos and videos, posting them all over their social media feeds. That is totally fine—for them. I don't want to ever be reminded of this particular day in my life.

Emma was allowed to take just one photo and I made her promise to never show anyone. I didn't look at the photo.

"It shows off your good cheekbones," Emma said.

I didn't look in the mirror while the very kind hairdresser

sensitively shaved my head. She didn't let any hair fall on the ground. It all went straight into a Tesco carrier bag so that I wouldn't get upset seeing the sad remnants scattered over the floor.

It took twenty minutes. I left the room with a beanie hat, soft against my new, unfamiliar, slightly-sore, stubbly head.

Once home I still didn't look in a mirror. Nor did I do so for eight whole days after the trip to the hairdresser. I was battling through the chemo side effects during the week of the head shave—recovering from the chemo train wreck that I am now sadly accustomed to dealing with every three weeks. I didn't have the emotional or physical strength to look in the mirror and cope with what was going to look back at me.

My wonderful children, my caring husband, my angel mother and my darling sister were super. They all lovingly stroked my newly bald, but still slightly stubbly, head and said exactly the right things.

"Mummy, you don't really look any different. You just don't have any hair," the children said that evening when they crept into my bedroom to look at this new person in their lives.

Yet again, my children made my heart burst.

I've looked in the mirror now. I did it a few days ago. I did it slowly and I hardly recognised the person looking back at me. I thought that I was prepared for losing my hair. I wasn't. Losing my hair has made me look completely different and I feel ugly. It has changed who I am on the outside and that makes me feel different on the inside. It emphasises the feelings that Breast Cancer has brought.

I feel vulnerable and ill. I'm like one of those cancer patients looking out from the posters and leaflets at the cancer centre information desk. I feel like losing my hair has made me take the inevitable step towards helpless, fragile cancer patient, and I'm pretty certain that along with my bird's-nest hair, a huge chunk of my self-confidence went into that Tesco carrier bag at the hairdressers.

CHECKLIST

Losing Your Hair

- Not all chemotherapy will cause hair loss so check with your oncologist.
- It's worth thinking about your hair options before starting chemo so you are prepared when your hair starts falling out.
- Find a local salon which provides a discreet service for ladies going through chemo to have their head shaved.
- If you are going to shave your head yourself, be careful not to cut yourself (remember your low immunity, you don't want to get an infection).
- Ask the hospital about using the cold cap if you are keen to keep your hair. It's worth trying it and seeing if it works for you. Lots of hospitals provide this now and there are things you need to do at each appointment (like wetting your hair and putting conditioner on it). For more information on using the cold cap look at the links on www.tickingoffbreastcancer.com.
- Think about whether you're going to get a wig.
- Ask the hospital if you will be given a wig.
- Look online for wig salons near where you live.

- Take a friend to a wig-fitting appointment. A friend sees your hair from all angles and can give honest advice about how much a wig looks like your original hair—if you're trying to replicate your own hair, that is.
- Get a wig liner made from a soft fabric because the underside of the wig can be uncomfortable.
- Special hair care is necessary while your hair starts to thin and throughout treatment if you are using the cold cap:
  1. Don't wash it every day.
  2. Use gentle shampoo and conditioner—pH neutral is good.
  3. Don't use styling products like mousse, gel or hairspray.
  4. Don't rub your hair with a towel. Blot it dry.
  5. Don't use a hairdryer, straighteners or heated curlers.
  6. Don't have your hair treated or coloured.
- Get a few scarves. These are a really comfortable way to cover your head.
- There are online tutorials to help you tie your head-scarves. Pinterest and YouTube are good places to start.
- There are also a lot of places selling hats which look like scarves but are already tied.
- Look for natural, soft fabrics because your scalp will be sensitive.
- Get a couple of nightcaps because sleeping with a bald head can be uncomfortable and cold at night.
- Check out www.tickingoffbreastcancer.com for places where you can buy scarves, hats and wigs, plus links to scarf-tying tutorials.

CHAPTER 10

LOSING CONTROL

"She's strong but she's exhausted."
R. H. Sin

We're already in cold, dark, grey February. One month of the New Year has passed already. Life continues and this week's to-do list goes something like this:

1. Do an online food shopping order.
2. Clean and tidy the house.
3. Pick up dry cleaning.
4. Do the washing.
5. Change the bed sheets.
6. Make a lasagne for the freezer.
7. Book the car in for an MOT.
8. Buy cards and gifts for all birthdays coming up in the next month.
9. Go through all the school admin from the past two weeks.
10. Pay credit card bill.
11. Put the garden furniture away.
12. Forget everything on this list and curl up under a

blanket to watch the box set of *Game of Thrones* because I feel so tired and rubbish thanks to the ghastly chemo.

Yep chemotherapy. I'm having chemotherapy because cancer cells were found in my lymph nodes, which means that they had spread there from somewhere else. The chemo is targeting any other cancer cells which may have escaped the 'original tumour'—well, they had to come from somewhere—but weren't caught when I had my lymph nodes removed. Plus, if there is a miniscule tumour in my breast—which, remember, was one of the possible scenarios—the chemo could shrink that down to, well, no tumour.

So, I am fully aware that I should be thankful to the chemo for blasting any evil cancer cells that may be secretly floating around my body.

My chemo routine goes something like this. . . I go to hospital every three weeks, on a Tuesday, to have my bloods taken. This is a regular blood test: a needle is inserted into a vein in my arm and enough blood is extracted to fill three small test-tube-type vials. Despite trying very hard, I'm still not doing well with needles and I still need to look away and hold my breath while the nurse does her business with my veins. If I'm lucky I get Linda taking my bloods—lovely Linda who held my hand during the biopsy of my armpit lump just four months ago.

I have rubbish veins in my right arm—where they take blood from—so I do everything that I can to help:

1. Drink plenty of water in the couple of hours before the blood test.

2. Pump my fist to get the blood moving.
3. Keep my arm warm.

Despite taking these steps, you can guarantee that my arm won't play ball and give up the blood easily. If Linda is on blood-taking duty when I arrive, she always groans because she knows she'll have a fight on her hands getting blood from me. In fact, she's been known to give up on me. This means that going for bloods on a Tuesday can take quite a while.

Gina or Libby usually come with me. They won't take no for an answer when it comes to taking me to medical appointments and, actually, it's a good excuse for us to get together; their chat provides a great distraction from the needle on blood-test days.

The hospital tests my blood for all sorts of things. There is a huge list of things and all of it is in medical code. The tests are essentially to check my general well-being, but all I'm told is whether my bloods, or 'neutrophils' to use the medically-correct word, are 'high enough' to undergo chemo the following day.

I know this means that I need to have enough healthy white blood cells to cope with the chemo. If this type of blood cell drops below a certain point then I will have to delay chemo until they are back up to the right level. So far, I haven't dipped below the cut-off point, which means I am on track for getting through chemo in accordance with the original timetable. I don't want any delays, thank you very much.

On Wednesday, the following day, I go in for my chemotherapy or, as I like to call it, my being-pumped-full-of-poison-therapy. I've noticed that some people get all dressed up for chemo. It's their way of defying cancer and showing that it can't control them. I totally get that and good on them. I, on the other hand, have become very fond of, what one might call, lounge-wear and the au naturel look. I even have a pair of boots which could be described as outdoor slippers.

The thought of putting on proper clothes and makeup just to go and be pumped full of poison just doesn't float my boat. I think that once this is all over, I might have a celebratory bonfire and burn all my chemo clothes.

My husband, Mum, Emma, Libby or Gina take me to chemo and they stay with me for the duration and give me a lift home. Sometimes I doze off; sometimes I'm quite chatty; sometimes I like to listen to a relaxation recording.

As I've said, there are a number of different chemotherapy drugs for breast cancer. The drug that I'm having at the moment is called EC. This is a combination of two chemotherapy drugs: Epirubicin and cyclophosphamide. It's a red liquid and it makes my wee red. Yes, really.

When I arrive at hospital, the first thing that happens is that I'm weighed. I get to see how much weight I've put on since last time. Contrary to what one might expect of a cancer patient, I am not losing weight, but gaining it, thanks to a combination of the medication, lack of my usual exercise routine and the rubbish that I am eating (shhh, don't tell anyone).

A nurse checks my blood pressure, oxygen levels and looks me over to ensure that I am doing well enough to have the chemo. No chemo is allowed if I am feeling poorly in any way.

There are various ways of administering chemotherapy drugs intravenously into someone, which means the drugs are pumped directly into a vein. They can be given through a cannula in the inner elbow, via a tube in the upper arm (a

PICC line) or via a tube into the neck or chest, which is called a central line.

I have the chemo drugs injected through a port in my chest just under my right clavicle. The port is a little box about the size and shape of a pound coin, out of which a tube feeds into a vein in my neck. The port and tube are hidden under my skin. I can't see anything by looking at my chest other than the faint outline of the port under the skin and the small scar from the incision. The port and tube were put into my chest under sedation and a local anaesthetic the day before my first chemo session.

It wasn't the nicest experience but, continuing with my trying-to-be-brave attitude, I think I dealt with it fairly well. I don't recall much of it other than talking an awful lot once they had injected me with the sedative, but I can't remember anything I said. I hope it wasn't too embarrassing.

To actually get the chemo drugs into the port, a nurse inserts a needle through my skin into the centre of the port. The first time a nurse did this I jumped out of my seat and the nurse missed the port. Since then I have applied EMLA cream to the skin over the port. It's a local anaesthetic and numbs the area, making the needle insertion much less uncomfortable. The needle is attached to a long, narrow tube, which is hooked up to a bag, like the drip bags you see in hospital dramas on the TV. With an array of tubes and leads and wires leading to and from a small beeping machine, about half the size of a shoebox, the liquid contents of the bag are slowly pumped into me via the port. The flow of the liquid is so slow that it drips rather than flows.

First, they pump through some steroids, anti-sickness

medication and antihistamines to help prevent sickness and allergic reactions. Then they get to the actual chemo drugs.

At my first chemo session, I was slightly concerned by the heavy-duty aprons that the chemo nurses wear when they attach the bag of chemo drugs to the IV. If they have to protect themselves so dramatically from inadvertent splashes of chemo drugs, what on earth are the drugs doing to my insides? They finish off with some more steroids and anti-sickness medication. In between each drug, a saline liquid is flushed through to clean the tubes. It is fairly time-consuming. The whole IV process takes around three hours.

Going to the hospital for chemotherapy isn't too bad in the grand scheme of things. There are, of course, a number of aspects that I don't like: the smell of the hospital, the churning in my stomach as I wait for my turn, the stab of the needle going through my skin and into my port, the coldness of the liquid as it first hits my veins, and the aftertaste in my mouth after I've had the drugs. But I do like the hospital vending machine's hot chocolate and the nurses.

I'm lucky to have such lovely chemo nurses. Roma is Scottish and has the most amazing accent I have ever heard; I could listen to her all day. She is also a whizz at taking blood. Vicky has a wicked sense of humour and has an answer to every difficult question that I ever ask. Jenny just walks into a room and before she's said a thing, we burst out laughing and Debbie—who seems to treat me more than any of the others—is kind, understanding and a total expert at distracting me and taking my mind off what we're doing. I don't know how they do it. They are consistently bubbly, upbeat and lovely. I now know what it means to describe someone as a ray of sunshine.

On the Thursday after a Chemo Wednesday, just as the nausea and side effects kick in and I'm feeling truly awful, I have to go back to hospital to have an injection into my stomach.

This injection, unimaginatively labelled by me as 'the Tummy Injection' helps my body to make more of the good blood cells, which in turn helps to raise my immunity level a little bit. Great in theory, but hard in reality. It has a HUGE, spring-based needle and it hurts as it goes in. It also makes me feel awful; headaches, swollen glands, aching all over like I have the flu, but it does an important job, so I have to get over it. Unlike some cancer patients, I don't have to do the Tummy Injection myself. Some people even have to give themselves an injection every day for a week or so after each chemo infusion.

I am given some steroids and anti-sickness medication in tablets to take at home for the few days following Chemo Wednesday. If I take the steroids after four o'clock in the afternoon, I'm awake all night. I've tried various combinations of anti-sickness medication but nothing takes away the nausea and I've become accustomed to feeling sick and nauseous for a good few days following chemo.

I worry about getting ill from the chemotherapy. Chemotherapy is given to increase the chances of survival from cancer but the treatment makes me feel so ill that I am concerned about whether some people die from the actual treatment itself.

Chemo works by, to put it bluntly, killing off the rapidly dividing cells inside the human body. It cannot differentiate between the nasty, rapidly dividing cancer cells and the good, healthy, rapidly dividing cells that your body needs. Whilst the chemo drug goes around blasting the nasty cancer cells, some of the good healthy cells get caught in the crossfire and are inadvertently blasted. Lots of lovely healthy cells like hair follicles, skin cells, cells in the gut, mouth and stomach, and ones that help with immunity all get caught out.

It's this blasting of my lovely, healthy, immunity-boosting cells that worries me. I feel so helpless against infection. It's been drummed into me that if my temperature goes over/under certain points then I need to go straight to A&E, but how can I possibly defend myself against all infections in the first place, especially as I have two young children? What else can I do other than be careful not to get any cuts or scrapes, and avoid anyone who's ill? What more can I do than carrying a packet of household antibacterial wipes and hand sanitiser with me at all times? Should I be greeting all visitors with a pump of antibacterial gel rather than a kiss and a hug?

It should be noted that my friends and I have perfected the art of the virtual kiss and hug. We may look a bit silly as we stand far apart, wrapping our arms around the thin air between us whilst kissing the air, but the thought is there! I mean, when else in life do you need a hug from a friend more than when you're feeling particularly shitty after chemo?

I've had three cycles of chemotherapy and each one has brought a longer, more intense period of side effects to deal with, because it turns out that the effects of chemo are cumulative.

Cycle one was administered ten days before Christmas and thankfully the worst of the side effects were over by Christmas Day, which meant we had the gorgeous, quiet family Christmas that we'd planned.

Cycle two was given to me on my forty-third birthday at the beginning of January. A birthday that I decided to cancel.

Normal birthday celebrations will resume once this detour is over. Cycle three was a couple of weeks ago.

Chemotherapy affects everyone differently: some people suffer a myriad of intense side effects whilst others have fewer and/or less acute symptoms. It all depends on the chemo drug, the dosage and ultimately the individual reaction of the person having it.

It seems to have hit me hard. Not that I really expected anything else, given my sensitivity to even taking a paracetamol. You hear of people going for chemo in their lunch hour, then returning to the office to pick up where they left off but it will come as no surprise that I haven't managed to return to work and that I've had to officially take an extended leave of absence.

Some people seem to be able to get out and about quite a bit, living as normal a life as possible and some people continue to run marathons, cycle the London-to-Brighton bike race, swim the channel and climb Mount Everest. Well, maybe not the last three, but seriously, running and cycling during chemo? Not me. I seem to slumber through two weeks of every three, battling the side effects, feeling awful.

In the days following chemo, my body does all sorts of strange things over which I have no control. I get incredibly hot, then incredibly cold; I have headaches and general aches and pains; I feel horribly nauseous and tired; and it feels as if every single cell in my body is quietly vibrating all the time. I even struggle with going up and down the stairs. I need a rest part way down and I often crawl, rather than walk, back up.

It's impossible to know which of these sensations is a normal reaction to the chemo drugs and which is abnormal when the normal side effects feel abnormal! I'm trying to get used to what is now normal for my body in this situation. This is where the traffic-light system comes in handy.

I've experienced plenty of the traffic-light side effects—those in each coloured section of my book. I've phoned the hospital for advice. However, not wanting to be labelled the 'oh-no-it's-her-again neurotic patient,' I'm reluctant to call them too often. So I have stumbled along with the assistance of a couple of helpful websites, common sense and the sound words of wisdom from my husband and mother.

I've been to A&E once. After one of my early chemo cycles, within a day of receiving the chemo drugs, I was experiencing horrible palpitations and breathlessness. It was scary. I phoned the hospital helpline and was told to go to A&E. Off I went for a raft of checks, tests and X-rays. It turned out not to be anything of concern like a blood clot, asthma attack or serious heart problem. In fact, the palpitations were just innocent, albeit unpleasant, palpitations.

It took longer than one visit to A&E for this diagnosis. I was referred by A&E to a cardiologist and I then had to wear a portable heart monitor for twenty-four hours immediately after the following chemo session, which was a right nuisance to say the least. My heart is fine. The palpitations are nothing serious and I have merely extended the parameters of what is now regarded as my normal reaction to these chemotherapy drugs.

With this chemo routine comes the chemo fog. Imagine being engulfed in a dark cloak and held in its tight grip so that you can't move in the same way you did before cancer. You're slower, shakier and clumsier. It stops your brain from functioning properly; you forget everything you're meant to remember. It plays havoc with your emotions: occasionally you're up, but mostly you're down, and all sorts of irrational and dark thoughts pass through your mind.

All my energy is now focused on getting through this treatment and recovering from the chemo train crash every three weeks.

The past two months have been a rollercoaster of palpitations, hot flushes, indigestion, heartburn, nausea, joint ache, back ache, mouth sores, an itchy sore throat, headaches, all-encompassing tiredness, brittle flaky nails, a non-stop dripping nose, pins and needles in my toes and fingers, a weird heightened sense of smell, sleepless nights, and let's be frank here and divulge everything—all sorts of gross, unpleasant changes to my bowel movements. My skin is red and sensitive, so with my bald head I resemble a tomato, and then there is the small matter of a complete shut-down of my mental capabilities.

I can't retain a darned thing in my head these days. It's called chemo-brain. It's an actual thing. They mention it in passing, as an aside, before you start chemo. Something they just throw in at the end of the chemo introduction meeting. The advice is focused on losing your hair: not losing your mind. Given the impact that chemo-brain has had on my life, I'm surprised that there was no big warning with flashing red lights. Or maybe there was? Thanks to my chemo-brain I can't actually remember.

Some say that chemo-brain is down to the 'fatigue and stress of cancer.' It's more than that:

1. *You may have changes in your memory, concentration, and ability to think clearly and put thoughts into action.'* YES.

2. *'You may be less organised than usual.'* YES.
3. *'And less able to focus.'* YES.
4. *'Or have trouble finding the right words.'* YES.
5. *'And with finishing sentences.'* YES.
6. *'Or lose your place while reading.'* YES.

Add to this the complete blanks that follow me around all day. I lose time. I forget entire conversations. I know I walked upstairs with that pile of clean washing but I have no idea where it is now. Seriously. . . where is it?

I'll retrace my steps time and time again. I'll concentrate until the cows come home, but from the point when I walked upstairs with it in my hands until now. . . a complete blank. Then maybe in a day or so whilst looking for something else that I've lost, I'll find it, usually somewhere like inside one of the kitchen drawers or the cupboard under the stairs.

The children laugh at me. They tell me things but then later, I have absolutely no recollection of our conversations. At least they're laughing.

This reduction in my mental capabilities is freaking me out. I used to be incredibly organised. Maybe even over-the-top organised. Control and I were the best of friends. I felt that in order to live my crazy-busy life I had to be on top of everything and that meant being completely and utterly organised. All. Of. The. Time.

I had to be organised at work, making the part-time arrangement work and proving that despite working part-time, I was still one hundred and fifty percent productive during my reduced hours. I also had to be organised at home, with the children, and in life generally.

During my crazy-busy life, lists were always my little bullet-point saviours keeping everything in line, controlling my life, allowing me to live that life and to ensure that it did not spontaneously combust and they worked. I was, most of the time, completely, efficiently, wonderfully in control.

Now, as I sit here writing out my to-do list for my good week, wrapped up in a warm blanket whilst a winter storm causes chaos outside, I'm shocked at how my life is so different from just a few short months ago. My life seems out of control in many ways. I couldn't control the cancer growing or spreading inside me. I have very little control over the treatment plan I am currently undergoing. I have no control over my body's reaction to the chemo drugs, nor whether the drugs will work. I can't control my completely over-the-top, crazy emotions or the irrational what-if wobbles that pop into my head. I couldn't control my hair follicles and I can no longer control my home because I feel too rubbish most of the time to clean, tidy, cook, iron, or do anything remotely useful. Control has most definitely departed.

I'm turning again to my little bullet-point saviours. Lists have become more important than ever before. Not because I'm juggling so many balls at once, but because I need to write down absolutely everything before I forget it. I have to rush to write down a thought before it evaporates into thin air. Sometimes there are only seconds between a thought forming and then it disappearing, so it's a frantic race to scribble it down or type it into my phone.

There isn't always something on which to note it down, so I have to repeat it, chant it or sing it out loud until I can write it down. The children and my husband are used to this raving lunatic rushing around reciting random words, sentences and phrases, scrambling for a scrap of paper or my phone.

"Send Granny's birthday card. . . Send Granny's birthday card. . . Send Granny's birthday card. . . Send Granny's birthday card. . . Send Granny's birthday card. . ."

"Muuuuuuummmmmm, I'm hungry. When's tea?"

"Ready in twenty minutes."

And that's enough for me to lose the thread and forget to send Granny's birthday card. I hate it. I hate that my brain won't retain the things that it used to. That it's slowed down and is now functioning at something like ten percent of its capacity.

Along with my hair, Breast Cancer has taken away the control I held over my life. It has taken away my ability to organise myself, my family, my home, the simple ability to recall and my mind.

So, my message to Breast Cancer is to take itself and its thirst for all that is important to me and to get lost. Go. Be off. Disappear. Jump back down off my shoulder and be gone.

CHECKLIST

Dealing With Chemo Side Effects

- Always call the hospital, your oncologist or your GP with any concerns. Check with your chemo team when you should call the hospital about side effects.
- Invest in a good-quality, digital, ear thermometer. You will need to call the hospital if your temperature goes above or below certain points.
- Keep a daily journal after each cycle of chemo, recording all side effects so you can compare how you feel after each cycle. You'll see if something is different from usual and you can ask your chemo nurses about it.
- Different chemo drugs have different side effects. The Cancer Research UK website has an excellent resource, which lists each of the breast cancer chemotherapy drugs and provides information on common, occasional and rare side effects, and what to do if you have them (see Appendix).
- Try not to worry or get stressed about the side effects because that will make you feel worse.
- Online forums and Facebook groups are an excellent place to ask other breast cancer patients for their

suggestions and tips on how to alleviate side effects (but always remember that other people may have different side effects to you).

- Remember that the side effects will pass eventually. Some of the cancer support organisations have helplines, using which you can chat to a nurse about any concerns. Have a look on www.tickingoffbreastcancer.com for links.
- **For sleep problems,** try some relaxation techniques including meditation, meditation Apps, regular bedtime routine, long soak in the bath. . . try what you can!
- **For a sore mouth:**
    1. Get all sore throats checked out by the hospital.
    2. Use a soft toothbrush and gentle toothpaste and mouthwash.
    3. Eat soft foods.
- **For nausea:**
    1. Try wearing travel sickness bands. But only on the arm that's okay and not the one lymph nodes have been removed from.
    2. Try some relaxation techniques.
    3. Ask your chemo nurses for more/different anti-sickness medication.
- **For taste changes,** try eating different foods.
- **For constipation,** ask the chemo nurses for a laxative recommendation, drink plenty of water, and eat fresh and dried fruit.
- **For loose bowel movements,** talk to your chemo nurses and oncologist.
- **For aching joints and bones,** ask your nurses and

oncologists. They may advise that you do a little bit of exercise every day such as a couple of short gentle walks.

- **For fatigue:**
  1. Exercise.
  2. Relax.
  3. Eat healthily.
  4. Drink plenty of fluids.
- **For dry and/or sensitive skin:**
  1. Moisturise all over every day.
  2. Choose gentle skincare products like body wash, moisturiser, face cleanser, moisturiser etc for sensitive skin.
  3. Use sun cream with a high protection factor.
- **For indigestion and heartburn,** check with your chemo team what you can take with the regime you are on.
- **For discoloured and/or ridged nails:**
  1. Use a hand cream.
  2. Use a nail oil or moisturiser.
  3. Keep nails short and well maintained.
  4. Wear gloves for washing up and gardening.
  5. Consider avoiding manicures and pedicures during chemo. This is to avoid the risk of infection from unclean implements or cuticle cuts. Remember your low immunity and possible risk of lymphoedema.
  6. Avoid nail gels and acrylics because they will weaken the nails and sometimes bacteria can get between the nail and the coating, causing infection.
  7. Use a non-acetone-based nail polish remover.

8. When on some chemo drugs, wearing dark nail varnish helps protect the nails because it provides a barrier between the nail and sunlight. Check with your chemo nurse if you are on one of these drugs.

- **For pins and needles in fingers and toes** (neuropathy), tell your chemo nurses/oncologist, so they can keep an eye on it.

CHAPTER 11

A GREAT-SHAPED HEAD

"Oh, I am very weary, though tears no longer flow; my eyes are tired of weeping, my heart is sick of woe."
Anne Bronte

I may not be used to the effects of chemo brain but I'm actually getting used to having no hair. No hair anywhere at all on my body. Well, actually, I have about three or four eyebrow hairs above each eye, which are holding on for dear life and I'm trying everything to keep them there. Other than that, it has all gone. From my head, my legs, even the soft downy hair on my arms has gone. I've lost hair from places I never even knew I had hair like in my nose! Now there is nothing to keep the snot and blood from just flowing freely out of my nose and onto whatever I happen to be holding at the time. And I can tell you, there is quite a lot of runny stuff that runs out my nose at the moment.

All the worrying about losing my hair before chemo started was focused on the hair on my head. I didn't give a thought to the hair everywhere else. I have to admit that I'm not keen on the no-eyelash-no-eyebrow look. Together with my puffy face and reddening skin, I don't look good at all.

However, I'm now feeling better about my bald head. Even the little stubbly hairs have fallen out. All that rubbing and scratching of my itchy scalp has worked the remaining stubble out of the follicles. My morning routine has been cut down significantly. It is wonderfully exhilarating. I wash my head with shower gel in the shower and then just moisturise it. I read up on what helps with the dryness and the itching. Slathering it in olive oil was one suggestion, but I smelt like a salad and the smell followed me around all day, so I haven't done that again.

I actually have a wig. She's called Brenda. Although perhaps a little bit tight, Brenda is amazing. She makes me look like the pre-cancer me. Brenda has been welcomed into our home by my children. She's been played with, dressed up and shown off to all our visitors. Admittedly, she also spends a lot of her time sitting on a polystyrene head on my dressing table attracting dust.

After the head shave, I found a little wig salon in the back roads of a town near me. I sent the hairdresser some photos of me and my lovely brownish-blond, wavy, shoulder-length hair so that she could find a selection of suitable matches. Then one Saturday afternoon, Libby, Emma, my daughter and I went for a fitting. The lady running the salon was wonderful. She had selected around ten wigs of a similar colour, length and curl to my natural hair.

The four of us sat while she got them out of their boxes and passed them around for us to look at and get a feel for the hair. Each wig had a name. They weren't 'short brown bob' or 'longish slightly blond one' or 'the one with the highlights.' They were Maggie, Sylvia, Frances and Pamela. Try keeping a straight face at that.

After a couple of hours trying out the wigs, plus a subsequent visit back to the salon a week later to have my chosen one cut and styled, I walked out looking exactly like pre-cancer me and went straight out to lunch with friends to celebrate the arrival of Brenda in our lives. It's unbelievable what a hairdresser can do with a wig.

I don't want to look like I have cancer when I'm doing anything that doesn't involve just resting at home, so I wear the wig out and about. Brenda is beautifully sleek and she looks amazingly similar to my old hair. With her on my head I can pass as normal i.e. not a bald cancer patient.

Despite looking like the old me, I don't feel like the old me and wearing a wig takes a bit of getting used to. It's weird. Unlike real hair, which is attached to your head, you can't tell when the wig is wonky or sitting the wrong way, making you look dishevelled and off-centre. You're really conscious of this—constantly wanting to look in a mirror to check that everything is straight. Plus, wearing a wig is hot. Really hot. The strands of hair are tightly woven into a mesh cap, which doesn't allow your head to breathe. The combination of this warm thing on your head, your body heat—which is heightened thanks to the chemo side effects—and the worry/embarrassment/stress at wearing a wig, but not wanting to look like you're wearing a wig, can often create much discomfort.

Then there's the tightness of the wig. It's not like wearing a hat. For some reason I thought it would be and the wig would just sit on my head. Oh no. It's got to be of a certain tightness so it doesn't:

1. Blow off.
2. Slide off.
3. Slip.
4. Slide down.
5. Get accidentally pulled off.

With the combination of heat, anxiety—mostly about what it looks like—and tightness, it sometimes feels like my head is in a vice. So much so that I am always popping to the toilet where I can sit down, pull off Brenda and relax.

I don't wear my wig, a scarf, or a hat around the house much at all. It's strangely invigorating. My husband says he quite likes it, although I strongly suspect that he's just being kind. The children don't even register that I look different now. Occasionally, we might talk about it, but they tend to say things like, "It's you now Mummy and we love you the way you are," or "You're still Mummy inside."

Even when people come over to visit, despite me looking strikingly different, the bald head doesn't get mentioned. Everyone seems to be used to the bald head now. When it was mentioned at first, most people said such lovely things, like:

"You suit a bald head."

"You have the features to go bald."

"It shows off your eyes."

"You have a lovely shaped head."

"You look like Sinead O'Connor."

I'll take all those compliments, thank you very much. I know that they would say these nice things even if my head looks odd, even if I don't have the features to carry off a bald head, even if my ears stick out, even if it doesn't show off my eyes, even if I don't have a great-shaped head, and even though I certainly don't look like Sinead O'Connor! They are very kind to say such lovely things and make me feel comfortable to be around them with my bald head on show.

Along with the rather striking change to my head, I'm also a bit red and puffy in my face and heavier all over. Steroids, and the medication generally, are clearly contributing factors to these changes, but I suspect the heaviness is a lot to do with the carb-fest that I am gorging on every day and it turns out that the menopause causes weight gain. Yes, I am well and truly in the full thrust of an intense menopause.

When I was diagnosed with breast cancer I had absolutely no expectation that going through treatment would kick-start the menopause for me. It just didn't cross my mind. The menopause is something that old women go through—silently, stoically and without making a fuss. I'm forty-three years old, which is certainly not the typical menopausal age.

Mr Oncologist mentioned at our first meeting that due to the type of breast cancer I have and the drugs I'm being given, there was a good chance that I might go through it. I was told to expect it to be an intense menopause because it would be an induced menopause rather than a natural one. Oh, Breast Cancer, you really are the gift that just keeps giving!

In addition to the abrupt halt to my periods in December, I'm now experiencing some delightful menopausal symptoms, which are, in all likelihood, also partly due to chemo:

1. Hot flushes.
2. Night sweats.
3. Tiredness.

4. Weight gain.
5. Memory lapses.
6. Crazy emotions.

Crazy emotions. Now that is an understatement. My emotions are up and down, back to front, inside out and all over the place. I don't know whether I'm coming or going. For someone who's usually a fairly level-headed person and has never experienced monthly mood swings, these are all out of character and really rather unpleasant. Along with Sadness, who's been an on-and-off fixture lately, Anxiety has now made an appearance.

Anxiety: that quiet, gloomy, all-encompassing, nagging, lingering emotion that is reluctant to let go once it gets a hold of you.

There's something about having cancer that invokes some sort of expectation on the patient to be brave, to fight and be inspirational, but this is impossible and actually I would say, unnatural. I often feel dreadful.

Daily life focuses on; getting up or sometimes not getting up; dressing, which mostly consists of baggy, lounging-around clothes; putting one foot slowly in front of the other as I shuffle through the day, often accompanied by tears and anxiety; and then going to bed. Repeated the following day and the next. This is not brave or inspirational: it's fearful and weak and boring but people don't want to hear this, so I tell them:

"I'm doing well. Tired, but doing well."

"It's fine really, just a few days of feeling awful after chemo, but then that settles down."

"I'm alright, thanks for asking."

"It's okay, really."

"Don't worry, I'm doing okay."

But what I don't say is:

"I feel truly awful and I can't stop crying."

"I can't stand having chemo."

"I'm really struggling today."

"I didn't get a wink of sleep last night because all I could think about was dying."

"I am so scared that this will kill me."

"I'm so sad that I can't come out with you this evening for the tenth time in a row. I miss going out and I'm so upset that I am missing out. Again."

"I am so jealous of you and your carefree life where the biggest decision is where to go on holiday next summer."

"I'm fed up."

"I cannot explain how utterly awful it is to get a cancer diagnosis."

"I can't breathe properly today."

"I hate being bald. I don't look good in any shape or form and I resent the fact that you've all got hair."

"I know that I should be feeling positive, but I don't feel that today."

"Why am I the one with breast cancer? It's so bloody unfair."

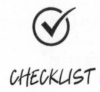

CHECKLIST

How To Alleviate Menopausal Symptoms

- Acupuncture, but not in an arm where you have no lymph nodes. Check with your oncologist if you can have this during chemo.
- For night sweats, keep a small can of water spray next to your bed, have a fan in the bedroom and use a 'chillow,' which is a cooling pillow.
- The menopause impacts your bone density over time and can lead to osteoporosis. To help prevent this, the advice is to ensure you have enough vitamin D and calcium in your diet. Check with your GP/oncologist about whether supplements are suitable for you. You may wish to consider taking advice from a specialist nutritionist about which supplements would help.
- Do gentle weight-bearing exercise. Check with a professional if you have had recent surgery, are now at risk of lymphoedema, or are having cancer treatment.
- HRT is not recommended for ladies who have had breast cancer.

CHAPTER 12

SCONES WITH CREAM AND JAM

"Food, like a loving touch or a glimpse of divine power, has that ability to comfort."
Norman Kolpas

We are still in gloomy February and it's a miserable day today. Big fat raindrops are pelting down the windows and water is gushing from the gutters onto the driveway. The roads are completely awash. The trees in the garden are swaying in the wind. The sky has fallen down and it looks like evening, even though it's only just past lunchtime.

Just like the damp, grey mist hanging around outside today, the chemo fog is still well and truly covering me; I can barely get from the bed to the lounge today. I am having a rest on the sofa, watching TV and writing a shopping list to text to Gina.

She, like Libby, has been doing an awful lot to help and support us: delivering home-cooked meals, taking me to scans and chemo, texting and phoning me regularly, keeping me sane, letting me bend her ear, and giving me a shoulder to cry on. Today, she's offered to collect a few things from the supermarket because I'm not up to leaving the house and my husband is working.

My shopping list looks like this:

1. Fresh pasta.
2. Crisps (preferably cheese-flavoured Kettle Chips).
3. Vanilla ice cream.
4. Cheddar cheese (preferably mature).
5. White bread.
6. Baked beans.
7. Potato waffles.

Gina doesn't recognise me from my shopping list. She double-checked that this was the right list. Where's the spinach? Blueberries? Wholegrain bread? Healthy soup? I don't even recognise myself. I used to eat healthily, but that's gone out of the window, along with a lot of my old ways. My eating habits have changed beyond recognition. Let me explain how my twenty-one-day chemo cycle goes in terms of my bizarre, new, eating habits.

Day One: Chemo Day

I usually eat a normal lunch at the hospital and then I eat plenty of snacks during the day. When I get home from hospital—before the nausea kicks in—I make a cup of tea and a cheese and coleslaw toastie. It's become a ritual. I get home and climb onto the sofa with a cup of tea and a toastie. A delicious, gooey mess of white doughy bread, crispy on the outside with the yummy scrumptiousness of melted cheddar cheese and crunchy coleslaw on the inside. It's just a little touch of heaven on those drab chemo days. Then, I'll have a normal dinner, but dinner absolutely has to involve a lot of stodge of some description, such as pastry, chips or mashed potatoes.

Day Two: I Always Feel Dreadful

I generally stay in bed, lying as still as possible in a quiet room, other than a quick trip to hospital for the Tummy Injection. Due to my non-stop nausea and difficulty in lifting my head off the pillow, I don't eat normal meals but I have small frequent snacks such as frozen orange juice pops, ginger tea, celery with peanut butter (I know, weird, but who knew it would be one of the very few things I could stomach whilst in a chemo slump), crackers and cheese, and plain biscuits. It's not so much a case of eating for enjoyment, but more of a case of trying to get some sustenance while trying to quell the nausea with food.

Day Three: Repeat Of Day Two

This is generally a repeat of Day Two but I'll eat a little more of everything.

Day Four: Feeling Slightly Better

This is when I start to feel slightly better. The nausea calms down but the effects of the Tummy Injection kick in. I'm usually able to move from the bed to the sofa. I'll go for a walk but that is usually the extent of my activity. However, this day usually marks the turning point of my appetite and I need to eat and to eat a lot. This is when I start to crave and eat the beige, bland, carbohydrate-heavy food.

Days Five to Fourteen: Gradual Improvement

I feel a little better every day during this period and eat everything that I can get my hands on. I can't stop eating everything that is bad for me: pasta, pies, pastry, buns, cakes, crisps, cheese, chips, chips with cheese, mashed potatoes, roast potatoes, boiled potatoes, and lots and lots of white bread—anything that is beige really.

I can't stand the thought of salad and vegetables. I certainly can't look at them, let alone eat them. I don't want to eat fish. I want to eat succulent red meat, preferably with stodgy pasta or melt-in-the-mouth pastry: lasagne, spaghetti bolognaise, beef stew and dumplings, steak pie, roast beef and roast potatoes.

I don't want to have healthy, hearty vegetable soups. I want to eat toasted cheese sandwiches, pies, quiches, crisps, chips, and baked beans.

I don't want to eat fruit. I want to eat cakes and buns and scones with cream and jam and lots and lots of milk chocolate. Not dark chocolate, which, at least, has a few antioxidants, but big bars of soothing, delicious, milk chocolate.

Days Fifteen to Twenty-One: I Feel Much Better.

This is my good week. I'm back to three meals a day (instead of four or five) and I don't have the cravings for stodge that accompanied me for the previous ten days.

This is so out of character for me and I'm well aware that I'm not following the guidance about having a healthy diet during chemo. I don't usually have a sweet tooth. I love vegetables. I love fish. I eat red meat maybe once a month. I eat salad every day. I love to eat healthily. Of all the times in my life when I should be eating as healthily as possible, I cannot bring myself to even look at a vegetable, or something wholegrain, without feeling nauseous.

I have a couple of lovely breast cancer cookbooks. I bought one at the start of chemo, and another one was a Christmas present. They look lovely and are filled from cover to cover with healthy, hearty, filling meals to help me through my cancer treatment, providing just the right nutrients and minerals to help my weakened body endure this tough chemo period. But I just can't bring myself to make any of the meals, or worse still, eat them.

This is yet another way in which the treatment is changing me. The steroids and the chemo have taken away my healthy appetite and replaced it with this bizarre desire for carbohydrates, red meat and sugar. I have come to the conclusion that if I'm to eat, then I need to go with what my body tells me to eat and when. During my bad weeks it is telling me to eat carbs and to eat them fairly regularly.

I'm eating to quell the nausea. I'm eating to give me the energy to get out of bed and to recover from the effects that the chemo has on every healthy, normal cell in my body. Maybe a little part of me is also eating for comfort.

So, with Love and Support keeping me company this afternoon, I won't feel guilty about tucking into scones with clotted cream and jam as I press play on the final season of the *Downton Abbey* box set that I am storming through during this cycle of chemo.

CHECKLIST

Eating During Chemo

- I couldn't face eating a number of healthy options during my chemo, but the advice is to eat as healthily as possible and there are a lot of helpful resources online. Also have a look at www.tickingoffbreastcancer.com or any of the websites listed in the Appendix.
- To avoid the risk of food poisoning, wash fruit and vegetables carefully, steer clear of un-pasteurised dairy products and takeaways.
- Check with your oncologist before taking any dietary supplements, even if you were taking them before diagnosis.
- Tips for eating to help with the nausea:
    1. Eat little and often.
    2. Try ginger things like ginger tea, ginger biscuits or stem ginger.
    3. Try peppermint tea or mint sweets.
    4. Try snacking on dry, plain food like plain crackers, water biscuits and dry toast.
    5. Boiled sweets can help.
    6. It is often a case of trying and seeing what works

for you in keeping the nausea at bay so go with what your tummy tells you.

- Eating to help with a change in taste and a furry, sore or metallic mouth:
    1. If you can eat pineapple, freeze small chunks of fresh pineapple in a freezer bag. These are great to suck on when your mouth feels grim.
    2. Make fresh fruit juice ice lollies using plastic or silicone lolly moulds.
    3. Use plastic or bamboo knives and forks if metal ones emphasis the metallic taste in your mouth.
    4. Avoid spicy foods such as curry and chillies.
    5. Avoid hard textured foods like French bread.
    6. If you don't fancy or can't eat solids, then have soups, smoothies, stews and juices.
    7. Ice cream or sorbet can be soothing for a sore mouth.
- Drink plenty of fluids. If water tastes horrid then try adding fresh fruit, a little squash or try drinking herbal teas.

CHAPTER 13

A FUNNY OLD DAY

"Sometimes life will kick you around, but sooner or later, you realise you're not just a survivor. You're a warrior, and you're stronger than anything life throws your way."
Brooke Davis

Every day is different with chemo and I suspect that in addition to this being down to the way I physically feel; this also has a lot to do with the hormonal imbalance and chemical fluctuations going on inside my head. There are good days, bad days, positive days, hide-under-duvet days, panic days and emotional days. In fact, going through cancer treatment is all about taking it one day at a time. Not thinking ahead, not planning. Just getting through the current day: ticking off the treatments, the side-effects and the medical appointments.

Bad Days

These are the days immediately following my chemo appointment when the drugs are coursing their way around my body, making me feel physically rubbish with the onslaught of chemo side effects. Days when the horrible chemo fog descends and I wonder how long it'll be until it lifts again. I spend most of these days lying in bed, waiting and hoping for sleep to take me away from the nausea and discomfort. Thanks to the steroids, which are meant to help ease the nausea, sleep is a rare commodity and I mostly end up just lying as still as I can, listening to the birds outside, as I try to focus on something to distract me from the sneaky whisperings of Fear and Anxiety.

Good Days

Not to be confused with Positive Days—which are days when I can bring myself to look forward to the future —Good Days are when I don't feel physically ill from the chemo. Perhaps a little tired, but good. I don't need to lie in bed or watch TV all day. I feel well enough to go out, to enjoy the fresh air and have lunch or a coffee, visit a friend, go to the gym and generally potter about getting on with the regular routine of normal life as a wife and mother. Breast Cancer still hangs around up on my shoulder, but, on the whole, I can happily get through a Good Day and dare I say, enjoy it.

Positive Days

Positive Days go one step further than a Good Day. They are days when, with Hope by my side, I feel particularly confident about getting through the treatment and coming out the other side. I feel sure that I will be cured of breast cancer and that this whole experience will just become a mere blip in my life. I allow myself to make plans for the future and I dare to think about things to come: birthdays, holidays, home improvements and even the children growing up. I particularly like a Positive Day.

Hide-Under-The-Duvet Days

Gloomy, grey, rainy days. These are different to the Bad Days because they don't just occur when I am feeling physically rubbish. They can hit at any time, out of the blue. They are the days when I cannot cope with talking to anyone. When I don't feel like putting my brave face on, pretending to be positive, discussing my treatment with a fake smile, or trying to be normal when clearly everything is so far away from normal.

These are the days when I just want to be left alone. Days when the tap won't shut off and I can't stop the overflow of tears streaming down my puffy, red face. When I feel resigned to the fact that I am a stupid cancer patient and I want to stop pretending everything is going to be alright and just wallow under the duvet with Sadness for company.

Panic Days

These are not good at all. This is when my heart beats faster, my palms are sweaty, tension hangs in the air and all I can think about is that I'm being treated for cancer. There's a party up on my shoulders on Panic Days: Breast Cancer, Fear, Anxiety and Sadness all whispering away to me, making me wonder whether I'll get through the treatment in one piece. I start to panic that the cancer has spread beyond my lymph nodes and that the treatment won't work in mopping up any stray cancer calls. I stress about whether the cancer will come back once treatment has ended. I can't eat or sleep. I can't focus on anything. On these days my heart constricts, the butterflies in my tummy are in supercharged mode and my mind goes crazy with thoughts and fears.

Emotional Rollercoaster Days

These are a bit of a mix of all the other days put together. I feel fine, then I'll feel scared, then positive, sad, worried, then back to good, then normal, thankful and then I feel rubbish. Breast Cancer hangs around, Fear and Anxiety usually make an appearance, Hope comes and goes, Love and Support might turn up, and Sadness often visits. So exhausting and unpleasant.

What kind of day was it today? Well, it was interesting. A funny old cancer day, one might say. Today was my first cycle of a different chemo drug after completing all six cycles of EC. It is called paclitaxel or Taxol. Most people, including Mr Oncologist and the chemo nurses, have said that Taxol is a less harsh drug in terms of side effects compared to EC.

I now have to go to hospital once a week to have this chemo drug administered—not like the EC chemo which was given to me once every three weeks. I need to do this for twelve weeks, which right now sounds like an awfully long time. It will be summer by the time I finish and it's only the beginning of March now. The good news is that I no longer have to go back on a Thursday for the Tummy Injection which is a massive bonus.

Back to today: my first paclitaxel. It all went well during the chemo session. I arrived as usual. Mum had driven me to the hospital and was my chemo buddy for the day. When we arrived, she had a coffee, I had my usual hot chocolate. We had to wait for a while today. It seemed to be one of the busier days when everyone had a chemo appointment at ten o'clock on Wednesday morning. I didn't mind waiting. I didn't really have anything better to be doing. It was a chance to chat to Mum, but as usual we ended up watching daytime TV during the waiting period.

Chemo appointments are, to be honest, the only times during this no-working, stay-at-home period of my life that I actually watch daytime TV. During my TV days at home when I can barely get out of bed or off the sofa, I'm usually working my way through a box set. On chemo days—thanks to daytime TV—I can catch up on celebrity news and gossip, check out the latest fashions, watch a couple go house-hunting in Australia, see a reluctant father being presented with the results of a paternity test, get a recipe or two, and generally re-join the rest of the world for a few hours. It's a great distraction from what's about to happen.

We went through the usual process: weigh-in, blood pressure, temperature check, oxygen check, IV in, pre-meds pumped through, new chemo drugs pumped through, post-meds pumped through, flushing the tubes, IV out and within six hours we were done.

I had to wait for longer than usual in the chemo ward after the infusion had finished today so that they could, ironically as it turns out, check I didn't have an allergic reaction to this new drug. All was well so off we went to get into the car to go home, but just as we were walking to the car, my top lip felt a bit peculiar: dry, swollen, soft, odd.

"Mum, my lip feels a bit odd. Does it look like the start of a cold sore?" I asked as we walked out of the automatic double doors at the main entrance.

We stopped and Mum examined my dodgy lip. "Well, it does looks dry and red and swollen."

I bent down to look in the wing mirror of a car.

"It feels really weird. What do you think?"

"It could be a reaction to the new chemo drug. Maybe you're having an allergic reaction?" she said.

Allergic reactions are fairly common in the world of chemotherapy. If an allergic reaction occurs as a result of the chemo drugs, you are pumped full of antihistamines and steroids, and depending on the severity of the reaction you are either moved to a different chemo drug, or given extra antihistamines and steroids before each chemo cycle. Because such reactions are not uncommon, you are constantly reminded by the nurses to report any unusual activity in your body.

Although everything feels rather unusual most of the time these days, Mum did think the lip swelling was more unusual than the usual unusual things. So, off we went, back into the chemo ward, just to be sure.

The quick diagnosis from the nurses confirmed an allergic reaction. They quickly rallied around, hooking me back up to the IV with lightning speed and pumping all sorts of things into me. I didn't want to be having an allergic reaction. I wanted to be at home.

"I'm sure it wasn't a reaction. It's just sore lips so nothing to worry about. Maybe it's the start of a cold sore?" I told the nurse.

And then the fire alarm went off.

Nurses were rushing around trying to administer the antihistamines and steroids; a doctor had been rushed down to the ward to check me out; I was insisting rather loudly that I wasn't having an allergic reaction so could I please go home; the fire alarm was going off; and it was a bit of a commotion really.

We had to evacuate. Evacuate sounds rather dramatic. We had to leave the building. Puffy, bald, tired, full-of-antihistamines-and-really-rather-woozy me, my IV, my pump, and all my tubes had to hobble along the corridor, leave the building and go out into the car park in the rain. Somehow someone had popped my coat over my shoulders. A chair and duvet were on the way. You really couldn't have made it up.

With hindsight, it was fairly amusing, but I remember the looks I got from people as they filed past me out of the hospital and into the car park; sadness, pity, concern. I was in my most raw state of cancer at that point: hooked up to my IV, woozy from all the antihistamines, bald, red, puffy, dressed in unattractive (yet comfy) tracksuit bottoms and sweatshirt, and moving incredibly slowly.

I was a portrait of cancer. I usually try very hard to hide my cancer-ish-ness when I'm out of the house: my wig, hat, makeup and regular clothes. Today my cancer was on show for all the world to see, which brought it home to me: I looked like one of those photos at the information desk that had I walked past at the cancer hospital before treatment started.

Oh crap, I realised, *I am now well and truly a cancer patient.*

CHECKLIST

Getting Through Treatment

- Be a *patient* patient.
- Take it one day at a time.
- Don't put pressure on yourself to do anything that you're not up to doing.
- Say no to things.
- Rest, rest and rest.
- Ask for help and accept help when it is offered.
- Talk to a partner, friend, family member or counsellor.
- Seek help from a support group if you need it.

CHAPTER 14

NIGHT-TIME CONVERSATIONS WITH BREAST CANCER AND FEAR

"Every night her thoughts weighed heavily on her soul but every morning she would get up to fight another day, every night she survived."
R. H. Sin

I'm lying in bed in the middle of the night, completely wide-awake, with no hope of sleep. Perhaps it's the effect of the steroids or the pesky palpitations? Maybe it's one of the other delightful side effects preventing sleep? It could be the March rain pounding on the windows and the wind whistling through the teeny, tiny crack between the window and the wall? Or, perhaps it's Fear and his pal, Worry, keeping me awake?

Night-time can be a mixed blessing for a cancer patient. Some nights are like this: awake during the dark hours with little hope of sleep. Other nights, I can be so incredibly tired from treatment that I fall into a deep, comforting, rejuvenating slumber.

There are times that I sleep so well that upon waking in the morning I forget that I'm bald and going through treatment for breast cancer. I have a few blissful seconds in which I'm normal again. I even reach for a hairband on the bedside table to tie back my long hair before I get up. . . and then it hits me.

Tonight, is not a night for sleeping. No, it's a night for conversations with Breast Cancer, Fear and Worry, as they dance around on my pillow. These conversations—my thought processes—tend to follow a pattern:

1. Being the natural worrier that I am, I worry about everything and anything. I still have all the normal worries of a forty-two-year-old woman and mother of two.

   Is my son unhappy about not being picked for the football team? Is my daughter sad because another girl was mean to her at school? What am I missing at work? Will I be able to go back to work?

   Of course, now I have the extra cancer worries to contend with, which basically all boil down to worrying about dying. The thing about dying that scares me most is not so much that I would miss out on stuff, but leaving the kids. I absolutely cannot bear to think how they would cope with their mother dying whilst they're so young.

   Mr Breast Consultant may have given me a good prognosis, but that was in the cold light of day, and thinking about my prognosis in the middle of the night is an entirely different story and I'm often joined by my what-if wobbles.

   Brain: "So, here we are again, Sara. No point in thinking about the future because you have cancer and you are going to die."

Me: "No I'm not. Mr Breast Consultant said he aimed to cure my cancer, which means I'll get through this."

Brain: "Well, of course he'll say that, but don't forget that there's still most likely a little tumour in your breast, which could grow and then spread and then kill you. So, let's plan your funeral. What music do you want?"

And so on.

2. I process, or rather I *try* to process, why Breast Cancer happened to choose me. Why did it come knocking at my door? Why did I, at the age of forty-two, get breast cancer?

I followed the rules. I did everything I should have done to avoid ever being in this situation. For goodness sake, I've drunk green tea and kale smoothies for years. I followed the freaking rules! Yet here I am. I mean, come on, how can this actually be happening to me?

What did I do wrong? Did I get stressed too much? Did I get my knickers in a twist about everything and create the wrong sorts of chemicals in my body that fed the cancer? Should I have eaten organic food? Did I not exercise enough? What could I have done differently so as not to be in this situation?

3. I analyse the bigger picture. I now realise that it's deceptive to think that we have control of our lives. That if we do the right things, like eating healthily, exercising, and taking care of our bodies, and don't do the wrong things, like smoking and frequently eating red meat, then we will live long and healthy lives.

We may think that we are in control, but in reality, we're not. We're not in control of our destinies. We're not travelling along a defined road, but along one with bumps and forks and detours and diversions and dead ends. At the end of the day, nobody knows where they'll end up.

4. I mull over mortality and survival. I think about how we can suddenly, thanks to something like a cancer diagnosis, be forced to look mortality square in the face. Until a life-threatening situation occurs, we don't think about when we're going to die. It doesn't register in our daily thoughts. We just naturally assume that we have endless time in which to do all the things we want to do: take the kids to Disneyland, ride a hot air balloon over the Serengeti, trek up a mountain, learn to sail, paint a masterpiece, write a book and, well, simply get old watching our children grow up. I mean, that's the natural order of life, isn't it?

Then, one day, out of the blue, your whole world can change. You suddenly realise the fragility of your mortality and you can think of nothing other than survival.

5. I muse over the loneliness of a cancer diagnosis. It can be incredibly lonely at times going through breast cancer treatment. As you will recall, I left normality and entered cancer-land on the day I was diagnosed with cancer and for a while now, I've been looking in on normality from my new vantage point, high up in this parallel universe of cancer-land.

I can see that life has pretty much carried on as

usual. My children continue to go to school and my husband, friends and colleagues go to work and about their day-to-day business. The earth keeps spinning, day turns into night, night turns into day, and life in normality continues as it always has.

Meanwhile, here I am in cancer-land and it's a lonely place. Yes, of course, my husband, family and friends have rallied round and could not have been more supportive but, none of my very close family or friends have ever had cancer. Some of them have known someone with cancer. A couple of them have sadly lost friends or family to cancer but they've never had it. They haven't experienced the shock of the diagnosis, the terror of the tests, the prodding, the poking, the scanning, the sleepless nights, the inability to eat, the heavy weight on their chest, the difficulty breathing, the constantly sweaty palms, the shaking, the anxiety, the worry or the fear. Despite them trying to help me in every way that they can, nobody can relate to how I'm feeling, or what I'm going through, and this is lonely.

You can have all the love in the world directed your way, but strangely, you can still feel the loneliest you've ever felt.

6. I reflect on what's important to me. Before Breast Cancer landed, my life had become so busy and so chaotic that I think I lost sight of the things that are really important to me: family, love, kindness, integrity. Four simple things which got pushed to the curb during all the rushing around.

I mean, yes, I see my parents regularly but it's always

when they're picking up the kids or rushing over to help with a burst pipe; it's not usually quality sit-and-talk time.

I love my children with all my heart, but we get so caught up in the constant rush of school, activities, homework and clubs. I have to ask: when do we just spend time *being* with each other? Let's not even try to work out the last time my husband and I had an evening out, just the two of us.

If I'm brutally honest with myself, maybe I'm guilty of caring too much about what other people think of me/my home/my clothes/my life rather than focusing on what I think of these things. This treatment has forced me to slow down, and by slowing down I have a lot of time to think about my life and assess whether it's what I want. Am I being true to myself in the way I'm living my life? And you know what? Things are definitely in need of change round here.

7. This may be a cancer-cliché, but I try to figure out some sort of reason for all of this happening. Cancer is frightful and there's nothing about cancer that makes me thankful for having it, but being a glass-half-full girl, I am trying to make sense of my current situation. Surely, being put through all this crap has to mean *something*? It has to be more than just a question of dodgy genes, malfunctioning cells, shit happens and bad luck?

I'm not saying that there is some higher power at work here, punishing me for some long forgotten/ non-existent sin or teaching me how to thrive in the face of adversity. Nor am I saying that everything in life—the good and the bad—happens for some divine reason or that I need to turn this into a positive experience. No, none of those, because having cancer is not any of those. However, a cancer diagnosis is so huge that I don't think I can just get through the treatment, move on and leave it behind me. I think I need to take it and use it somehow. Not allow it to just invade my life for no reason.

I can get very busy in the pitch black of night, asking question after question, rarely coming up with any answers and constantly searching for peace of mind. It is exhausting but not exhausting enough to bring sleep tonight.

CHECKLIST

How To Relax

- Relaxation techniques you may wish to try are:
    1. Meditation: the practice of calming and focusing your mind, using breathing with the aim of creating inner peace.
    2. Mindfulness: the practice of being present in the moment and switching off from all external distractions.
    3. Hypnotherapy: a form of therapy that uses the power of positive suggestion to bring about subconscious changes to our thoughts, feelings and behaviour.
    4. Guided relaxation: involves listening to a soothing voice telling you to imagine yourself on a lovely beach, relaxing every part of your body, and before you know it, you're fast asleep.
    5. Reiki: a practitioner places their hands on your body to unblock the life-force energy within you that has become stagnant.
    6. Reflexology: a therapist will apply pressure on

and massage, different points on your body, which is thought to help alleviate symptoms.

7. EFT tapping or Emotional Freedom Technique: with the help of your EFT therapist, tap various parts of your hand, face and shoulder whilst saying a personal mantra to alleviate a particular anxiety or phobia or general feelings of stress.

- Sometimes, when everything is just a bit too much and you can't bring yourself to even listen to a soothing voice telling you to relax, you might like to search YouTube and try listening to relaxation music or relaxing white noise.

- You can try replacing negative thoughts with positive affirmations and keep repeating the affirmation until you feel better. An affirmation is just a short sentence or statement such as, "I accept the chemotherapy drugs into my body, so that they can help my body fight the cancer cells."

- Cancer support centres often offer some of these relaxation techniques.

- There are plenty of online relaxation resources and Apps.

- www.tickingoffbreastcancer.com has links to plenty of relaxation resources.

CHAPTER 15

THE IMPORTANCE OF BEING DISTRACTED

*"You may never know how strong you are until being strong is
the only choice you have."*
Bob Marley

I'm listening to a Radio Four afternoon play. The quintes-
sentially English voices have a soothing quality about them
and they're keeping me company on this grey, chilly, Tuesday
afternoon at the end of March.

There's something relaxing about being wrapped up in
a blanket on the kitchen sofa listening to the sounds of a
radio play, drinking tea while heavy rain pours down outside.
Sometimes, my mind tunes out and I miss what's going on,
distracted by the whispers of Breast Cancer, Fear, or one of
my band of little companions, but it doesn't matter if I don't
follow the play; it's just the soothing nature of the Radio Four
voices and the background sound effects of the countryside that
I like. I can drift away and then re-join them, leaving Breast
Cancer and Fear behind for a few blissful moments.

Chemo has been continuing its same unpleasant path of
weekly Taxol infusions. Despite the mini allergic reaction, I
haven't been moved to a different drug. I get more antihistamines

and steroids, which seem to do the trick because nothing has happened since the first cycle. Just as I was told, these chemo drugs are not as hardcore for me as the first lot. They bring some, but not as many, side effects. Thankfully. I count my lucky stars because I've come across some women for whom this drug has been worse than the others, which just goes to show how chemo drugs affect everyone differently.

I've also started having my Herceptin injections. That's the biotherapy drug I have every three weeks for one year, which works by attaching itself to the HER2 receptors on any stray cancer cells, so that they're no longer stimulated to grow.

These injections are, it must be said, a bit of a walk in the park compared to chemo for me. Although that may not be the case for everyone. One of the nurses injects the Herceptin into my thigh over the course of a few minutes to make sure that it doesn't sting. Other than having to see a cardiologist every twelve weeks for an ECG to check that the Herceptin is not damaging my heart, that's about it, really. I'm seeing the cardiologist anyway because of my palpitations, so I don't mind these extra appointments.

I'm still off work. It's a little odd not working. Clearly, I'm not up to going to work, but I miss the people, getting out of the house, doing something that I enjoyed, and the routine that work gave me. It also means that I have a lot more time on my hands.

My routine is now based upon hospital appointments and where I am in the current chemo cycle. I tend not to plan ahead too much at the moment because I have come to realise that if I plan something, I can't guarantee that I'll feel well enough to do it. Whilst this is totally out of my comfort zone, because I like to live a structured, organised, well-planned life, it's actually quite nice. I mostly just see how I feel each day, and then see where the day takes me.

This combination of more time and less planning, means that I continue to have those pesky what-if wobbles, so I need a good distraction from all this cancer malarkey. Thus, I try to keep busy and distracted, which is quite difficult given that I have the energy of a flat battery and, thanks to chemo brain, my mind is working at approximately ten percent of its normal functionality. However, it turns out that I can fill my time quite easily. Even with these limitations I have a pretty decent menu of distractions from which to choose:

1. Resting.
2. Exercise, for example walking.
3. Watching TV.
4. Reading.
5. Planning house furnishings.
6. Relaxing.
7. Listening to the radio.

The first item on my list (which isn't really a distraction as such) is to rest and I have to admit that I rest a lot. I'm permanently exhausted and aching.

Early on during treatment, I gave into the fatigue and allowed myself to rest when I needed to. It was an unusual concept for me to get my head around and to stop feeling guilty about. I think that most women feel the same. Us women just can't sit down and do nothing. There's always something that needs to be done. Don't get me wrong, I know that men do a lot of stuff too, but bear with me while I go on about the pressures faced by women.

We have to manage the laundry basket, empty the bins, sort the recycling, top up the dishwasher with rinse aid, plan fun family activities for the weekends, change the bed sheets, clothe the continually growing children, scrub the toilet, book the car in for a service, keep on top of the family admin, and constantly work our way through the hundreds of jobs that are sitting on the endless to-do list of life.

That's not even including the expectations on us (as mostly set by ourselves) to have a career and/or worthwhile voluntary interests. Plus, importantly, the need to stay informed on environmental matters, political issues and world affairs generally. We push ourselves to look good, exercise, stay trim, and maintain a flawless face whilst trying to keep up with all the latest trends.

Furthermore, we have to do all of the above without complaining, getting ill, showing any signs of weakness, or generally losing it.

We just keep going and going, paying no heed to our own wellbeing or health. We are at the bottom of the pecking order. We give everything we have to making sure the family are looked after. Most of us do all this whilst working, whether full-time or part-time. We don't give ourselves a break! We keep going until something breaks us.

Something has broken me.

I feel broken, in so many ways, thanks to the chemo side effects. So, now, I'm allowing myself to rest, and to rest as much as I need. My place on the sofa has been assigned and I have a lovely assortment of soft blankets and scarves keeping me warm. I also have a fabulous collection of comfortable clothes, which are really rather suitable for lounging around on the sofa, and the slippers have, quite frankly, come into their own with all the lounging around that is going on.

The next distraction on my list is exercise. I've been told time and time again that exercise is really important during treatment, even though it's often the last thing that I feel like doing, so I'm making an effort on the exercise-front. I'm not a sporty type. I would love to be a sporty type, but those genes went to my sister Emma.

Throughout my early adult life, I tried various forms of exercise including: fitness classes, but I'm not really great with coordination; going to the gym, but I found that boring; and attending Yoga or Pilates, which I enjoyed but it didn't tick the cardiovascular-exercise box.

Not being a natural runner, a few years ago I decided I wanted to see what all the running hype was about so I did the couch-to-five kilometres programme. This is an App on your phone that talks you through a regular walk/run programme, building you up over a period of nine weeks. The goal is that at the end of the nine-week programme, you'll be able to run five kilometres. I achieved the goal, but it took closer to nine months. Not because I wasn't dedicated—I most certainly was—but because of my dodgy back.

Remember the booby MRI? To cut a long story short, my ability to exercise was hampered in recent years by my dodgy back and it turns out that running is one of the worst things to do when suffering from a dodgy back. A disc prolapse and facet joint degenerative wear and tear was taking its toll on me. However, in the nine months immediately before

D-Day, I was making great progress in recovering from my back problem.

I was seeing a rehab personal trainer and doing a combination of strength exercises, swimming two or three times a week and walking loads. The week before D-Day I happened to say to my personal trainer, "I'm feeling great. I can't remember the last time I felt so good." Ha bloody ha.

Surgery and chemo have seriously impeded my exercise regime. I'm not swimming because, quite frankly, I don't trust the germ situation at the local swimming pool. It's not the cleanest of places and whilst I used to just close my mind to that when I was going regularly, my immediate fear of any germs has put me off.

I'm still seeing my personal trainer, but not as regularly. More like when I feel up to it rather than every week. So, I'm left with walking. Despite being permanently tired, I try to walk every day, and sometimes twice a day.

Thanks to the encouragement (nagging) from the nurses, my mum and husband, I peel myself off the sofa, tie my trainer laces and put one foot slowly in front of the other. I can walk around the roads close to my house, but that isn't particularly appealing, so I generally take a five-minute drive to an old manor house. Once there you can imagine that you're in the middle of the countryside: there's a wide private road leading to the old house that's long since converted for some other use, surrounded by fields and woods. Not a road, car, lorry, shop or house in sight.

On the days straight after chemo, I can just about make three-hundred metres along the road and back, walking at the pace of a snail, unable to catch my breath with Breast Cancer and Fear pushing down on my chest, aching all over and the tingling quivering shaking feelings inside each cell within my body screaming at me to climb back onto the sofa.

On other days, I can walk much further.

I've come to love my walks. I've delighted in watching the seasons change from the hazy tail end of summer, when I was diagnosed, to a golden-brown autumn after surgery and on to the bitterly cold winter of chemotherapy.

Now, at the end of March, as I traipse along my usual route, I can spy the signs of spring. I wonder whether there is anything nicer than going for a walk just when we are on the cusp of spring? It's a time when the air no longer feels damp, cold and biting, but instead is becoming a gentle nothingness. Not cold nor warm, just still. I can breathe this beautiful air without it painfully piercing my chest with its icicle fingers. My shoulders can relax, no longer holding the weight of winter upon them.

The steps I take are lighter, less heavy, slower. I'm not rushing—as much as a lumbering chemo patient can rush—to get the walk over and done so I can return to the warmth of home, but instead I can take my time and enjoy the experience.

Instead of walking along with my head facing downwards in an attempt to avoid the piercing cold or driving rain, I can stand up straight and hold my head high, allowing the gentle, still air to touch my face; a face that was previously covered in scarves, protecting it from the winter chill. I still wear my hat over my bald head – that isn't ready to be exposed to the elements just yet.

Fields stretch out to the horizon, turning green as their crops begin to grow. Trees extend as far as the eye can see, not yet in full bloom but a hazy green from all the buds appearing on the branches. The sky is a beautiful cobalt blue, with wisps of white clouds floating around here and there.

Sometimes on my walks I have company; my husband, mum, the children or a friend. Someone to lean on as I stumble along the path. As lucky as I am to have the company, I also like being on my own here. I pop in my ear buds and listen to my uplifting, kick-cancer-in-the-butt playlist.

Coming back to the list of distractions, I mentioned that I watch loads of TV box sets and films. I love box sets. I can get through a box set or two per chemo cycle. I watch anything and everything: English period dramas, American crime dramas, thrillers and strange random shows, some with English subtitles.

I was invited to a party recently. I couldn't go because it was fairly soon after chemo day, a period during which I am in bed every night by eight o'clock and if I'd gone, I would have only had two topics of conversation to get me through the small talk: box sets and chemo side effects. Not really party conversations. Then again, I wasn't really in a party mood and I would rather have been at home with my box sets.

Fourth on my list of distractions is reading. I've always enjoyed reading. I love the way you can be completely transported to another time and place merely by some words on a page. Words can inspire your imagination and make time disappear while you join the characters of the story.

Soon after diagnosis, when I knew that I may be out of action for a while, I piled up all the books that I had been meaning to read but hadn't quite got around to: *The 19th Wife*, *The Tea Planter's Wife*, *War and Peace*, *Atonement*, *Mom & Me & Mom*, *The Light Between Oceans* and *The Miniaturist*.

When treatment began, I couldn't read a book. I couldn't stay focused on the page. My mind would wander even before I reached the second paragraph. It was no good. I kept having to re-read passages over and over again, losing the thread of the story. I think I must be feeling less anxious now because I can get through a book, fully absorbed in the story, and I now find it hard to put a good book down. Books make the days pass quickly, for which I'm thankful.

In addition to books, I'm completely addicted to home magazines and online home furnishing pictures. Given the time that I'm allowing myself to rest, I have time now to plan our house furnishings.

I've decided to make our home gorgeous. I'm going to paint this wall dark grey, get that chair upholstered in navy velvet, put a picture rail up for a gallery of black-and-white family photos, change the lamp shades, and create a cosy reading corner in our lounge. My house will be stylish, beautiful, ordered and wonderful. I have big, beautiful, soft, eye-catching plans.

Mostly, I just love looking at beautiful photos of beautiful rooms that look nothing like my home and that my home will never look like. Rooms that look out over the sea, a field, a lake or a river, that are full of wonderful colours and textures. Rooms with no clutter or mess.

What is it about a beautiful room that soothes me so? Maybe it's because it has absolutely nothing to do with cancer, health, hospitals or wellbeing? Maybe it's because these perfect rooms are so well ordered, clean, tidy and beautiful, which is a stark contrast to my home at the moment. Maybe it's because they represent hope? Something for me to aspire to once I am done with cancer.

Next on the list of distractions is to relax or at least I try to relax. Fairly early on in treatment, my nine-year-old daughter wrote me a letter with some advice.

Dear Mummy,
Ten things to do to get better:
1. *Relax*
2. *Relax*
3. *Relax*
4. *Relax*
5. *Relax*
6. *Relax*
7. *Relax*
8. *Relax*
9. *Relax*
10. *Hug me!*

Obviously, I was very proud of the numbered list, but the actual advice was really rather sound. I've tried a whole host of relaxation techniques in an attempt to relieve my aching body and soothe my frantic mind. Meditation, mindfulness, guided relaxation recordings, EFT (which is the tapping one), Reflexology and Reiki. I'll try anything to get me through this treatment.

As I mentioned earlier, I have a friend who created a personal guided relaxation recording for me. She takes me on a journey down some steps into a magical healing place where she gives instructions to my brain on how to switch off the side effects. I go to my main switchboard, locate the switch for, say, palpitations, and turn them off.

I don't know how effective it is, or whether my brain follows the instructions properly, but I do know that listening to a soothing voice against a background of gentle music has carried me through many of the worst days and nights of this treatment.

Sometimes, when I'm feeling truly awful and I can't get out of bed, when the TV, radio, audiobooks are all too much and when the silence is deafening, I listen to the birds outside in the garden. I open the window and focus on that faint, sweet, shrill sound just to get me through the day.

Earlier today I ventured to a cancer hospice for the first time. There's one near where I live, which is for people who are living with cancer. I didn't know such places existed. I naturally associated the word 'hospice' with end of life treatment, the thought of which totally freaked me out, so I didn't want to go. My GP friend suggested that I go and have a look at what they do for people like me, i.e. someone who's going through breast cancer treatment but isn't dying from it.

Antonia took me to make sure I actually arrived and didn't accidentally-on-purpose drive past. I was really nervous. Partly because I seem to have developed a mild form of agoraphobia and partly because it's yet another place for ill people— reminding me that I'm ill. But it was fine.

The hospice was a building all on its own, set back from the main hospital. The building itself was low, white and a bit like a bungalow. It was surrounded by beautiful greenery and flowers, which were clearly tended on a regular basis by a hoard of green-fingered volunteers. The gardens gave the place a we-are-not-a-medical-facility feel.

Inside, it was decorated in a combination of pink and purple soft furnishings with lots of wooden tables covered in magazines, books and leaflets. It was manned by a group of kind looking, middle-aged women wearing scarves and lanyards around their necks.

I had a cuppa and chat to one of the volunteers. It turns out that along with being able to drop in anytime for a chat, they put on all sorts of relaxing things like Yoga, Reiki and Acupuncture, for us breast cancer ladies. So, perhaps it was worth the visit after all.

Number seven on the list is listening to the radio. Usually Radio Four because of the talking. There is only talking on Radio Four. It's nice to have someone talking to you when you're the only one in the house day in, day out, with Breast Cancer and Fear for company.

I prefer the talking on Radio Four to the songs on the music stations. I still find that a lot of the songs on music radio stations have terribly sad lyrics which, given my current hormonal-ups-but-mostly-downs, make me cry. So, I mostly listen to Radio Four, but not the news, because that often makes me cry too.

With the help of these distractions, I pass the time. I'm slowly but surely getting through this treatment period and every day is a day closer to the treatment being over.

CHECKLIST

Distraction Suggestions

- TV box sets and films or consider subscribing to one of the online streaming TV/movie services.
- Exercise.
- See friends and family.
- Try crafts, knitting or sewing.
- Write. Write anything—a journal, maybe a poem or that novel you've always planned to write.
- Start a blog or website.
- Sort out your photos.
- Cooking. Make various meals to freeze for your rough days.
- Gardening.
- Plan to redecorate your home.
- Plan a holiday for when you're feeling better.
- Pinterest is a great place to look for things to do.
- Reading.
- Podcasts.
- Listen to audiobooks.
- Puzzle books, crosswords and mindfulness colouring books.

- Sort out some cupboards—if you feel up to it.
- Go outdoors. Whether it's exercising or just sitting, get out there. Fresh air, vitamin D and being around nature are all reasons for spending time outside.

CHAPTER 16

A KISS GOODNIGHT

"While we try to teach our children all about life, our children teach us what life is all about."
Angela Schwind

I'm trying to decide whether I can feed the children pizza or spaghetti bolognaise again for tea today. Those are the two family-meal staples on offer when I'm on cooking duty these days. Both require the least possible effort on my part. We have a lot of lovely bolognaise sauces in the freezer, donated by a host of generous, wonderful friends, and I have taken to stocking up on plenty of pizzas because they are so easy.

I am—as I have always been—the cook in our family because my husband is not home in time to help prepare dinner and cooking isn't really his thing anyway. But meals at the moment are a mishmash of donations from friends, my mum's cooking and the easiest meals I can put together. My domestic abilities have been severely challenged over the past six months. Control continues to elude me at home on many levels. Washing and ironing have taken a back seat. The house is a mess and there is always a pile of family admin a foot high to be worked through.

I feel completely out of control where the children are concerned. I'm not on top of what homework they have; which projects need to be done and by when; the days and times of their music lessons; practising their spellings and times tables; or who has a party to go to and when.

I'm finding it difficult to keep up with what's going on at school, the school play rehearsal timetable, the plans for the choir tour, who is playing in which sport team at which location, and I'm not really on top of what they are learning at school. However, I will shortly find out, because this evening is parents' evening at school for my son.

We've reached the end of the Easter academic term and I feel like I've slept though his entire time in Year Seven. I made it as far as October half-term before Breast Cancer made her appearance and, quite frankly, since then I've been rather distracted and, I hate to say it, self-absorbed.

I've tried very hard to still be a good mother to my children throughout the past six months but it's been very difficult. The combination of feeling constantly tired, tearful, ill from the rubbish side effects of chemo and having chemo brain have inevitably all had an effect.

However, whilst I may be travelling on a personal detour with Breast Cancer (and her entourage) by my side, I do realise that family life goes on and I have a constant to-do list following me around all the time:

1. Prepare meals.
2. Washing.
3. Ironing.
4. Clean and straighten up the house.

5. Sort out the bills.
6. Get on with all life's little jobs that need to be done.
7. Be a mum to the children.

Despite me being selfishly wrapped up in my breast cancer bubble, my children still need their mother. Importantly, they need to be listened to, heard, hugged and loved. Most importantly, they still need to be tucked up in bed and kissed goodnight at the end of the day.

Their lives need to carry on as usual, despite the arrival of Breast Cancer in our home. They still have to go to school, do their homework, make sure they take in a pound for the bake sale, see their friends after school and at weekends, go to Brownie camp and go to their clubs. We're trying very hard to keep everyday life as normal as possible.

It's been a challenge at times, but I've had plenty of amazing support from friends, for which I will always be grateful. Mum has continued with her pattern of staying with us for the few days following each chemo infusion. I have help with the school run, friends regularly have the children over after school and at weekends, and they are doing all the things that kids without a mum-with-cancer do.

I can get the children up and ready for school and muddle through the after-school period of clubs, homework, dinner and bedtime, albeit moving slower and forgetting a lot (chemo brain).

I'm aware that the children have fears of their own about my cancer so I'm trying to keep my ears and eyes open to any signs of stress or worry on their part. We talk about cancer quite openly at home. It's become a normal part of our lives.

They know they can ask me any question about cancer and the treatment:

"What happens when you go to hospital for your chemo?"

"When will you be better?"

"When will your hair grow back?"

"Can I feel your port?"

"Can I wear your wig?"

"Why do you have to go to hospital all the time?"

"You're not going to die, are you?"

The wonderful thing about children is their amazing resilience. Their marvellous ability to just keep going and get on with it. In fact, I sometimes think that my children have forgotten that I was recently diagnosed with breast cancer and that I'm going through some pretty tough treatment. A lot of the time they certainly don't seem to have changed their behaviour to accommodate me.

Whilst they are both good-hearted, lovely children who will get on with their homework, serve up their own meals, or bring me a cup of tea if I'm in bed, they still bicker and argue over who will have the first bath, what to watch on TV, who will set and clear the meal table, and everything that two children aged nine and eleven can argue over.

Like all nine and eleven year olds, they like to complain. They complain that "this bolognaise doesn't taste like normal bolognaise" or "this fish pie isn't your fish pie." They complain about not being allowed to have friends over to the house whilst I'm going through treatment. They complain that I don't take them to school on my Bad Days. They complain about doing homework.

Whilst I would appreciate more peace and quiet around the

house now and again, less arguing, and that they would do their homework without nagging, or eat tea without moaning, I love it.

I love the arguing, the bickering and the complaining. I adore the absolute normalcy of it all and that my two darling children are not really worrying about their mother but are just carrying on their lives as usual.

I like that their days are not defined by a mother having breast cancer and that they don't look at me in any different way now that I am completely bald. I love that they often comment that they can't remember what I looked like with long hair and that they think I'm cuddlier now that I've put on weight. They have never once said that I look awful or don't look like Mummy. I love that they are not aware of the seriousness of the situation and that life is carrying on for them in as normal a way as possible.

Their normalcy is infectious. I nag my children. I moan at my children. I tell them off but I also hug them. A LOT. I laugh with them. I cuddle them. I dance with them around the kitchen with my bald head bopping up and down to the radio, ignoring the man in the garden who is trimming the apple tree. I watch films with them. I watch TV with them. I play games with them. I talk to them. I listen to them. I hear them. I spend time with them. I love them.

I kiss them goodnight every single night. Even if it means them coming into my room where I'm already tucked up in bed as they go off to bed, when they lovingly stroke my bald head, hug me and kiss me goodnight.

CHECKLIST

Telling The Children And Helping Them Through Your Breast Cancer

- How you tell your children that you have cancer will depend on their age.
- Honesty is a good policy.
- Remember, you know your children best, so use your judgment as to how, when and what to tell them.
- The main cancer charities have excellent advice on talking to children about cancer (see Appendix).
- There are a lot of picture books which can help you to explain the situation to younger children. Have a look at www.tickingoffbreastcancer.com.
- There is a good selection of books to help tell older children and teenagers about your diagnosis.
- How to help your children:
    1. Try to keep life and routines as normal as possible.
    2. Tell the school about your diagnosis.
    3. Ask friends and school mums for help taking kids to and from school, clubs etc.
    4. Ask friends and school mums to have the

children at weekends, school holidays and after school when you need a break.

5. Take care of yourself. If you don't look after yourself then your recovery will be slow and it will ultimately impact the kids more.

6. Plan some nice family things to do at points throughout treatment, and at the end of treatment, so you all have something to look forward to.

7. Respect your children's feelings about your diagnosis and treatment.

8. Think of some ways to help younger children deal with the upheavals that treatment can bring. For example, for those low immunity days when your child is poorly and you have to keep clear:

    a. Give them a teddy to be your little helper and who can give out cuddles when you can't.

    b. Have a 'hug jar.' Every time your child needs a hug but you can't give one your child pops a token in the jar. Then, when you are around for hugs, he/she can count them up and call in the hugs.

CHAPTER 17

A TEENY TINY LITTLE IDEA

"Write hard and clear about what hurts."
Ernest Hemingway

It's a beautiful day today and I'm pretty sure that summer is just around the corner. We're at the end of May and it's blissfully warm. It's a lovely, gentle warmth, which slips in through the open windows at home, and brushes past me as I walk down the road and across the field. With the change from cold to warm, I've discarded my shawls and scarves. I'm no longer in need of fluffy slippers or thick socks. Instead, I'm enjoying the warmth reaching in and heating up my cold, achy bones.

Walking along my usual path, I notice that the trees are bigger, lusher, and full of leaves, buds and blossoms. The grass along the edge of the path is knee-high, the fields are overflowing with crops, the air is full of birdsong, the sky is bluer and blankets of wild flowers cover the verges. The days are brighter. And I am brighter because. . . CHEMO HAS FINISHED!

The most horrible six months of chemo treatment came to an end three weeks ago. Hooray! Yippee! Yay! Ya-hoo! Round of applause, please.

To mark the occasion, Gina and Libby visited me on the chemo ward with cakes for the chemo nurses and pink, bubbly, pomegranate juice for us, which we drank out of plastic champagne flutes pretending it was the real deal—it turns out that I can't stomach alcohol these days. Like all the milestones that I have reached, and will continue to reach during treatment, it was certainly a day to celebrate.

How do I feel about reaching the end of chemo? I know that I've constantly moaned about chemo, but now that it's over, I do appreciate what it's done in terms of mopping up any stray cancer cells and going towards preventing any recurrence or spread. I feel relieved, positive and hopeful.

I'm relieved that I no longer have to go through the actual chemotherapy infusion process; that the side effects should now start to improve; that I came through relatively unscathed without experiencing any truly awful effects; that I only had one trip to A&E; and that I no longer have to constantly keep track of my traffic-light system of side effects.

I'm pleased that my immunity will now increase and get back to normal so I can worry less about getting an infection. I feel positive because I'm another step closer to the end of treatment and thus to being rid of this cancer. I'm beginning to feel hopeful.

With the end of chemo, the chemo fog has lifted. Yay! It's been three weeks since my last chemo session and it's as if I'm now looking at the world in colour again. I feel significantly lighter and less shaky. I can move around more easily and walk a little bit further. I'm still very tired, but it's not the excruciating tiredness of chemo. Yes, I still experience some of the side effects of chemo, and I'm told to expect some of them to carry on for months, but everything is just clearer, focused, brighter, and much, much lovelier.

Part of the elation of ending chemo is that I have hair! Very short, stubbly hair. The hair on my head miraculously started to grow back halfway through the Taxol cycles. Tiny, dark-brown, hard, stubbly hairs have sprouted all over my head and I absolutely love it.

To add to the general furore and excitement of chemo finishing, I have a project now. I'm really quite excited by it. It started when Libby told me about her friend, Becky, who had just been diagnosed with breast cancer. Breast Cancer, why can't you just keep to yourself? Well, Libby asked if I could talk to Becky about what to expect from treatment, and really just be someone to chat to. Which, of course, I agreed to. Us breast cancer patients need to stick together.

There's an automatic bond with a fellow breast cancer patient—a solidarity between those who've experienced the diagnosis, the fear, the stress, the unknown, the anxiety, the waiting for test results, the medical appointments, the sleepless nights, the angst, the cold sweats and the dread.

Now, what would Becky need to know? She had been diagnosed but hadn't had any treatment. She was due to have surgery, chemo, radiotherapy, Herceptin and Tamoxifen. I could chat to her about treatment until the cows came home; it's all I know at the moment. My small-talk topic for parties could come in handy after all. However, I wanted to tread carefully. What would I have wanted someone to tell me when I was at her stage, between diagnosis and surgery? How did I feel when I was there?

I knew exactly what I would have wanted: practical tips. What should I take to hospital for surgery? What should I do about preparing for chemo? What should I expect from chemo? What should I take to chemo? What do I need to know about the cold cap? I didn't even know about such a thing until just before I started treatment. What should I do to prepare my home life for the treatment period? How could I alleviate the side effects? And a little, gentle, heads-up on what to expect from the aftermath of surgery and chemo.

I would have wanted a hand to hold mine and for someone to say, "It's going to be tough but you've got this, and to help you, here's what you can do to prepare. . ."

So, that's exactly what I intend to do and I'm not going to just do it for Becky. I want to do it for other people who've been diagnosed with breast cancer and are starting out on the turbulent road through diagnosis and treatment. I'm going to take all my experience, my shopping lists, my to-do lists, my checklists, all my resources and put them on a very simple, friendly, hand-holding website.

It'll be the one that I would have liked when I was diagnosed and first embarking on the breast cancer path, petrified about what I might find online. It'll be easy to navigate and not completely overwhelming, where you don't have to perform many clicks to get to what you need. A website without any photographs of bald men and women with cups of tea, talking to nurses, walking on a beach, gardening and holding hands with their significant others.

It won't mention anything about survival statistics, treatment success rates, the process of metastasis of cancer or the correlation between grades and stages and survival (there are plenty of other places to read about all of this online). Just helpful practical tips and advice.

I've come to realise that everyone reacts differently to their cancer diagnosis. Some people like to go on a fact-finding mission when it comes to their cancer, reading all the information they can find on their type of cancer, analysing all the clinical research, looking into drug trials, probing the statistics for survival/recurrence/spread, and investigating all the treatment options, whilst weighing up the pros and cons of associated success rates and side effects.

On the other end of the spectrum, there are those who are uncomfortable about reading up on, and researching, cancer and all the related information about treating it and surviving it.

Me? Well, so far, I have fallen in the middle of this spectrum and perhaps I've edged slightly closer to a burying-my-head-in-the-sand attitude. Back in normality (which you will recall I left on October 19th) the old me would definitely have been at the 'thorough research' end of the spectrum, but here, in cancer-land, I just haven't been able to bring myself to do it.

I can take on board what I've been told by Mr Breast Consultant, Mr Oncologist and all the other medical staff I've come across at various stages. I can ask questions and rely on the fact that Mr Breast Consultant has referred my case to his colleagues. I can research all the practical stuff but when it comes to looking for statistics about treatment success, spread and recurrence, I don't want to know (maybe for the time being, or maybe forever). It's almost as if knowing too much can take away hope.

I really want to grow old and be there beside my children as they grow up. I want to live my life to the fullest with my husband, sell up once the kids leave home and travel the world.

If I know too much about my chances of recurrence or developing secondary breast cancer—which I do know is the spread of primary breast cancer beyond the lymph nodes into other parts of the body and which is incurable—then maybe I'll be unnecessarily dashing those hopes. Thanks to my crazy hormones and the chemical imbalance caused by chemo, I'm so anxious as it is that I'm sure doing research on Google would just add to those worries.

I'm reaching into my heart where I wedged Mr Breast Consultant's good prognosis and that's all I need right now. I don't want to read the small print about my cancer.

We come to that cancer-cliché again, but maybe this website I'm building is what I have been looking for over the past few months. Something positive to take from all this utter crappiness. A way to pay forward all the care and kindness that I've received from so many people during my treatment. Maybe, part of the 'old me' is starting to peek through again. The research-driven, I-love-a-project, give-me-a-plan part of me.

Whilst trying to ignore Breast Cancer and her band of little soldiers who remain firmly positioned on my shoulders, I've pulled my head from out of the sand and started to look around a bit. I have bravely navigated the Internet and carefully sought practical information to enhance what I already know and I have found so much! There are endless support networks out there.

There are support centres, online forums, yoga groups, courses for every step of the way and online support groups.

There are websites selling products specifically for cancer patients: chemo care packages, special sweets to quell the nausea, bags for carrying around the drain after surgery (oh, if only I'd found these after my surgery), and clothing.

There are different types of clothing. There are clothes with easy access to the port for during chemo, clothes made from bamboo to absorb the night sweats and super-soft clothes for comfort.

There are charities which provide treats and days out for people going through cancer and their children. There are places that provide information about employment rights for someone going through cancer. Also, websites that help you to understand your treatment and provide the most useful glossaries of breast cancer terminology. There are online organisers to help you remember when to take your medication and plenty of motivational advice about exercising.

I've found YouTube tutorials for applying makeup to camouflage the lack of eyelashes and eyebrows, as well as advice about telling your children about your cancer diagnosis and how to reduce the risk of developing lymphoedema. There are booklets you can order or download on every breast cancer topic under the sun and there are a lot of blogs following the breast cancer experiences of many amazing women.

To continue with lifting my head out of the sand, I'm tapping into the Twitter breast cancer support community. I've also decided to join a Facebook support group, which is full of inspirational women—who funnily enough really don't like to be called 'inspirational,' which makes me like them even more! They are all going through breast cancer treatment and supporting each other every step of the way.

I'm going to brave another trip to the local hospice, which prides itself on helping people living through cancer and provides Yoga courses, Reflexology treatments and all sorts of lovely things to help those going through breast cancer. I'm going to download an App on my phone to help motivate me to exercise and I'll learn how to apply makeup so it looks like I have eyelashes, even though I don't. Plus, I'm going to order a couple of those booklets to read.

On my little, home-made, DIY website, I'm going to put signposts to every helpful thing I've found online and link to all the amazing, wonderful, practical resources that are hidden away in the vast cyber-universe of the Internet.

I'm going to write lists, tips and advice for every step of the way to help those who are embarking on breast cancer treatment but don't know where to go for help. Those who are standing at the edge of the breast cancer precipice not knowing which way to turn and are scared of what they may find if they look online for breast cancer support. It'll be for people who don't know that there's a treasure trove of wonderful support on the Internet and are scared to take a peek for fear of what they may read (which cannot be unread). It'll be for people who may need someone to hold their hand and say, "It's going to be tough but you've got this, and to help you, here's what you can do to prepare. . ."

If you're like me and you want to tick off the stages of breast cancer treatment as you go through it then I welcome you to www.tickingoffbreastcancer.com

CHECKLIST

Ways To Share Your Story

- Start a blog.
- Set up a website.
- Write a blog post for someone else's website or blog.
- Write an article for a cancer organisation's website or magazine.
- Share your story on Facebook, Instagram or Twitter.
- Write a book.

CHAPTER 18

I CAN'T REMEMBER IF I SHOULD BREATHE IN OR OUT

"I am not what happened to me. I am what I chose to become."
Carl Jung

I'm sitting in the kitchen, looking at the garden, with a cup of tea. Delicious, refreshing, peppermint tea, which I used to drink a lot and now that the wretched chemo is over, I can stomach again. The summer sky is a lovely clear blue with a few wispy white clouds dancing high up above the earth. The birds are chattering from tree to tree. Other than a little bit of traffic up and down the road, going past the garden now and again, it's fairly quiet here.

As soon as the chemo fog lifted, I moved away from the lounge sofa. The sofa was my constant companion during the endless weeks of tiredness, nausea, aches and pains; it was supportive, non-demanding and perfectly placed opposite the television.

With the end of chemo and the weather brightening up, I've felt a desire to be in the kitchen where the sun shines through our windows from sunrise to mid-afternoon, reflecting my generally brighter mood, and I can sit looking out upon the garden.

I'm still very tired and a few chemo side effects are lingering, plus I have the radiotherapy fatigue. I started the radiotherapy stage of treatment a week and a half ago, so I've been mostly sitting listening to the radio and writing for my website although I've been able to intersperse this with a little bit more housework, a bit of tidying here and there, following the odd recipe so that we are not stuck with pizza and spaghetti bolognaise, getting out and about, and gardening.

I've never gardened before. Until this year, we used to have a lawn surrounded by a few big shrubs. A minimal-effort garden, and one that didn't have much colour but I've become quite a potterer in the garden these days. It started as just going outside into the garden for a dose of fresh air and vitamin D. As I sat in the garden, gazing at our bare flowerbeds and empty patio, I started to picture flowers, shrubs, plants and pots. I moved away from the online pictures of beautifully decorated rooms to online pictures of gardens and, oh my, what a new world that is!

There are so many different styles of garden. Everything you could possibly think of. There are traditional English country gardens with trailing roses and wisteria, gardens full of every flower under the sun, and those with modern brickwork and minimal vegetation. There are gardens with vegetable patches and some with herbs. There are also some quite complicated instructions for planting things. You have to plant at certain times of year. Some plants are not suited to certain types of soil (and there are lots of types of soil). Some plants like sun and others like shade. The holes need to be dug to a certain size and on and on and on. Well, that's all far too complicated for my chemo brain, so I just potter.

Every day I try to pop out into the garden. Sometimes just for five minutes, sometimes for half an hour. Sometimes once a day, sometimes two or three times. We've become regulars at the local garden centre. Mum has given me some tomato plants, courgette plants and roses. She's also given me the advice I needed, because of course I don't know the first thing about gardens and plants. It's been lovely, kneeling side by side pulling up the weeds and chatting. We now have a few pots on the patio: roses, olive trees, hydrangeas and other plants and flowers (I have no idea of their names). At weekends, my husband has been planting our recent purchases together with the plant-gifts that we've received over the past few months: a pear tree and a couple of small roses. It's coming together.

My husband has always been good in the garden. He mows, he trims, he cuts, he digs, he tidies and he generally keeps the garden shipshape. In fact, along with a lot of turf-laying, he's also recently planted a wonderful, tall hedge of laurel trees next to the fence along the pavement side. He spent hours and hours digging and hauling and planting so that I could comfortably go out into the garden with my bald head without fear of being overlooked by the neighbours over the road. The hedge is growing magnificently—growing with all the vigour and vitality of my new hair.

One of the nicest things about having the kitchen doors wide open and spending a lot of time in the garden is getting the children outside after school and at the weekends. There's a ladder against the fence to our next-door neighbour's garden, and one on their side of the fence, so that the two little girls who live next door can climb over to us, and my daughter can climb over there. It's not unusual for me to turn my head from what I'm doing in the kitchen, or lift my head off the kitchen sofa where I've been napping/writing/reading/resting, to find all the children in the garden.

Just as my children are absolutely fine with my nearly-bald-but-now-there-is-a-fine-covering-of-new-hair head, the neighbour's girls have not given me a second glance either, which helps with gaining confidence about my new look.

The garden was a great distraction during the wait for radiotherapy to start and has continued to be a great distraction since radiotherapy started. I've found that Breast Cancer, and her chums Fear, Anxiety and Worry, tend to leave me alone in the garden. Instead, I am often joined by Hope.

I've now had seven sessions of radiotherapy out of a total of fifteen sessions. I have one per day, but not at weekends, which means I'll have the treatment for three consecutive weeks. So, I am essentially halfway through. Hooray. A few weeks ago I went for the radiotherapy planning session. At this appointment:

1. I had a CT scan so the team could plan exactly where they would be aiming the radiation. This involved me lying very still on my back on a table in a scanning room, while a radiographer moved me into various positions, scanning me at various points.

2. I had three tiny black dots permanently tattooed onto my chest (one between my breasts and the other two on each side of my chest where my bra strap would usually sit). These are to ensure that at each radiotherapy session the team can line me up in the same position each time. These are miniscule and just look like freckles.

Now, every day I arrive, I wait for my turn and go into a treatment room, take off my top, lie down on a treatment table, breathe in, get zapped, get dressed and leave. I spend, probably, around five minutes lying on the table with my boobs out, being manoeuvred into position by two nurses. Given events of the past eight months, I'm so used to taking my top off and my boobs being the centre of attention in a room, that I'm totally over any sort of embarrassment at being topless around strangers.

My son's teacher, the Mayor of London and a member of the Royal family could all walk in on me at this point, and, seriously, I wouldn't bat an eyelid. Using my three tiny dot tattoos as a guide, the nurses move my upper body and arms into position to the nearest millimetre to ensure that the radiation is aimed at the exact spot where it's needed. I'm then not allowed to move from that position, not one crucial millimetre.

Although the process of having radiotherapy treatment is easier for me than chemo, it does bring its own challenges. My left boob is being zapped and of course my heart is on my left side, just there under my boob. The radiotherapy treatment that I'm having requires me to hold my breath for the actual zapping to make sure that my heart moves out of the way. To do this, I have to wear what can only be described as a snorkel in my mouth (which holds my mouth open) and a peg on my nose. The snorkel is hooked up to a computer to monitor my breathing patterns. I wear goggles too, which are also hooked up to the computer, and all I can see through these goggles is the computer screen with the axis of a graph and various red and green lines.

As I breathe in, the red line goes upwards on the graph. As I breathe out, the red line falls down. Up and down. Up and down. Lots of little red triangles with the odd squiggle where I've attempted to swallow, which, seriously, is really difficult with a peg on my nose and a snorkel keeping my mouth open—go on, try it!

Whilst wearing this contraption and lying completely and utterly still, I have to hold my breath at three points during each session. First, for around forty seconds while the CT scan is carried out. Then twice more of around thirty seconds for each of the radiation zaps on my left breast.

The monitor on the screen in my goggles is to help me with that. I watch my breathing patterns on the monitor and when someone says to me through a microphone, "Hold your breath." I have to breathe in until the line on the graph reaches a certain point and then I have to keep holding it until I'm told to breathe out again. It is hard to hold your breath while your mouth is open. Thirty seconds is a very long time. Forty seconds is a very, very long time.

I started off by trying to do the forty seconds in one go. It was impossible, so now I break it in half and do two twenty-second breath holds. It's okay to do that for the scan, it just means I'm going through the process twice. I can just about hold my breath for thirty seconds, although I'm convinced that the clock on the goggle monitor is not right. Those seconds are much slower than the seconds I count in my head, '*One Mississippi, two Mississippi, three Mississippi. . .*'

At first, I got myself in a bit of a state. I was dutifully holding my breath and at around the twenty-five-second point, just before I was expecting to hear, "You can breathe normally again" through the microphone, I couldn't remember if I was going to have to breathe in or breathe out. It was as if I had switched off the breathe-button in my brain so when it was time to start breathing again, I didn't know whether to breathe in or out.

Along with starting radiotherapy, I've also embarked upon hormone therapy. This is a daily tablet called Tamoxifen. Remember, my breast cancer tested positive for oestrogen receptors? Well, Tamoxifen blocks the effects of oestrogen on these receptors, helping to stop oestrogen from encouraging any breast cancer cells to grow.

Tamoxifen is an innocent-looking, flat, circular tablet approximately eight millimetres in diameter. I take one at breakfast time every day.

When Mr Oncologist talked to me about how long I would be taking the tablets he said, "You'll take them for five years. Sometimes they're taken for ten years, but ten years is a long time in oncology."

I may forget a lot of what is said to me during my medical appointments, but I clearly remember that statement. Did he mean that ten years is a long time because of the constant advancement in medicine and what is prescribed today may well be superseded by a newer, better drug within the next ten years? Or did he mean that ten years is a long time because cancer patients do not often make it to the ten-year point?

In any event, I'm now taking my daily Tamoxifen tablet and I cannot say that I'm keen on them. I naively expected it to be like taking a vitamin tablet. I didn't expect the tablet to have any effect on me. I was completely wrong. They're not innocent little tablets at all. They make my hot flushes and night sweats about one hundred times worse than they were. Although I can't quite put my finger on it, they're making me feel even less like me than I already feel. I'm not sure how I'll cope with taking them for ten years (if I last that long, apparently).

Back to this beautiful sunny day. It's so calming, sitting here sipping my tea in the kitchen, as I wait to be collected by a friend who's driving me to my radiotherapy appointment. In fact, after all the hustle and bustle of chemo, I'm generally feeling much calmer these days. Radiotherapy is tiring but not as much as chemo and I'm not as stressed as I was during chemo. Things are looking up.

CHECKLIST

Radiotherapy

- Wear a non-wire bra, or sports bra, to prevent any friction from the wire causing you discomfort. Or don't wear a bra at all.
- Stock up on some good moisturiser for the area where you will be zapped. Your radiotherapy team will give you a recommendation.
- Apply the cream to the zapping area morning and night from a few days before you start radiotherapy, and every day throughout, continuing after radiotherapy until your skin has recovered sufficiently.
- Store your moisturiser in the fridge to give it an even cooler application.
- Use gentle, chemical-free soaps in the bath and shower.
- After showering and bathing, pat dry the skin at the zapping zone to prevent friction from causing your skin to get sore.
- You can't shave, wax, or use hair-removal creams on the armpit whilst you are going through the treatment. Remember to de-fuzz before your first appointment (if you wish).

- You will feel gradually more tired as you go through this treatment. Try to conserve energy where possible. A little bit of gentle exercise helps with the tiredness.
- Be prepared for your skin to get redder and sorer in the couple of weeks after radiotherapy, and for your tiredness to continue for a few weeks.
- If your skin gets very sore, you can get a barrier cream and soft cushioned dressings to protect it. Speak to your radiographers for advice if this occurs.
- ALWAYS ask for medical advice if your skin gets really sore, or something just doesn't feel right.
- You may feel well enough to drive yourself to and from radiotherapy appointments, but the tiredness does kick in after a week or so; you may want to ask friends or family members for help. Plus, the company to and from the appointments is a great distraction.

CHAPTER 19

HIDING IN THE SUPERMARKET FLOWER STAND

"The greatest healing therapy is friendship and love."
Hubert H. Humphrey

My daughter's friend, who is on a gluten-free diet, has come for tea. Of course, I don't have gluten-free food in the house. However, the sun is shining, I'm no longer doing chemo, I have a light covering of fine hair on my head (it's still the early days of hair regrowth but I'm getting used to holding my head up high and going out and about without a wig or hat), I'm just over halfway through radiotherapy and I'm actually feeling good, so I'm going to pop to the supermarket with a short list of basic items to buy for the perfect play-date:

1. Gluten-free sausages.
2. Gluten-free bread rolls.
3. Ice cream.
4. Ice lollies.
5. Sweets.
6. Chocolate.
7. Lemonade.

Going to the supermarket is a big deal. I've avoided the supermarket for a good while now. I've wanted to avoid the germs on the trolley handles, the stares at my wigged head or, God forbid, at my obvious chemo scarf, and the very well-meaning questions from the school mums, Brownie mums, Cub mums, swimming mums, football mums and cricket mums I'm bound to bump into. I have also been revelling in the joy of online food shopping and home deliveries, which, to me, is one of life's little miracles.

Today is a very hot June Saturday afternoon and I know that the supermarket will be quiet because I will have missed the morning BBQ rush and I'm too early for the afternoon BBQ replenishment rush. So off I go. I'm taking my time, pushing my trolley in the blissfully cool, quiet supermarket. I trundle down the ice lolly aisle when I look up and see her. The last person I want to see. For someone who can only lumber along these days due to the combination of a chemo cocktail, very little exercise, a dodgy back, cancer fatigue and flip flops, I'm surprised by how quickly I can do a one-hundred-and-eighty-degree U-turn out of the ice lolly aisle and into the perfect cover of the flower stand. I'm forty-three years old and I'm in the flower stand hiding from someone.

It's an old friend of mine. Let's call her Susie. How I know her isn't really important for the purpose of this little anecdote. What is important (well, to me anyway) is that after telling her of my diagnosis within a couple of days of D-Day, I had a text to say she was sorry to hear the news but I haven't heard from her since and that makes me very sad.

I realised early on during this experience that us human beings crave three basic things. Food and water of course, but there's something else we need: we have a basic need to know that we're cared about. It gives us a reason to exist. To be cared about is something we must earn throughout life, but when we have it, it keeps us going through thick and thin, through pain and suffering, through bad times and any of life's hardships. Being diagnosed with breast cancer is one of those bad times when knowing that you are cared about can help carry you along and deliver you out the other side.

I realise how lucky I've been with the love and support that I have had from my family, friends, acquaintances and even strangers. It has, without doubt, been my lifeline on this unenviable trip. However, there is something jarring about an old friend not getting in touch over the course of the past eight months. Eight months of scans, tests, stress, fear, surgery, drains, pain, physio, needles, bloods, anxiety, tears, hormones, chemo, hair loss, sadness, aches, injections, palpitations, sweats, terror, pre-meds, steroids, puffiness, fear, radiotherapy and soreness.

After much deliberation on this issue, I've come to realise that this situation is not unusual. Going through a traumatic life event will most likely show you who your friends are; there's a good chance that at least one friend will not behave as one might expect a friend to behave during your cancer treatment. It's a bitter pill to swallow, but it happens and it happens for a variety of reasons. Although there may well be the friend who's just a bit thoughtless and doesn't realise the magnitude of what you're going through, most of the time if someone isn't there for you, it's probably down to something more understandable.

Some people may find it hard to be around a cancer patient;

they just don't know what to say or how to act or what to do. Some people may be dealing with their own personal issues, of which you know nothing about, making it hard for them to be there for you, and some people may find that being around someone with cancer causes anxiety, fear or even opens old wounds.

My advice to anyone who can't (for whatever reason) be there for their friend who has cancer, please just acknowledge this and let them know. It'll save a lot of soul-searching and upset.

Back to me in the supermarket. I'm not ready to face Susie. I can just picture the conversation:

Susie: "Oh, hi. I am soooo sorry I haven't been in touch. I've been so rubbish."

Me: "Oh, don't worry. It's nothing. I'm fine. No need to worry."

You see, I have this need to put people at ease and to avoid any kind of confrontation. I hate awkwardness and any sort of unpleasantness. I smooth over all potential awkward situations. I suppose all of this goes hand in hand with being the natural worrier that I am, and the way I worry about what other people think. But I am not fine.

I'm really sad that I haven't heard from her. I'm not in a place to deal with this right here and now. So, if I pop on my sunglasses, I'm in perfect disguise. She hasn't seen me since before cancer, when I had brownish-blond, wavy, shoulder-length hair. I now have a very short, spikey, thinning, brown/grey combo, which is a bit patchy on the crown. And I've put on weight. I can get to the till, pay and escape without her seeing me and I do. I escape.

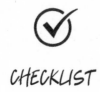

CHECKLIST

Your Friends

- Even though you don't want them to, people will treat you differently. That's just how it is.
- Ask for, and accept, help from your friends.
- Tell your friends how you feel so that they can try to understand. They could read this book.
- Tell your friends when you are up to going out and when you would rather not.
- Understand that some people say the wrong thing because they don't know what to say.
- You are not expected to repay favours while going through treatment.
- Don't take it personally if friends disappear.
- Cherish the friends who step up.
- You may make new friends through support groups and social media who are going through the same thing.
- Remember that you are loved and cared about.

CHAPTER 20

A CANCEREE'S TRIBE

"Close friends are truly life's treasures."
Vincent Van Gogh

Seeing Susie has made me think about this need to be cared about and my appreciation for the fact that I haven't had to get through this detour alone. I've had so many people with me on this diversion out into the wilderness of cancer-land—a tribe really. In addition to the vast quantities of love and support, people have brought many different things to this cancer party and I imagine it's similar for many people going through this experience, or even some other traumatic life event or illness.

I've found that, with their different personalities, friends have different ways of helping out, each stepping outside the comfort of their own lives and showing their best qualities, as they give practical help, emotional support and, above all, such wonderful kindness.

For me, my friends fall into one of the following categories. Some fit squarely in one camp whilst others have attributes which span more than one. Whilst I describe everyone in these categories as female—because my tribe was female—you'll probably find that male friends also fit these descriptions:

Practical, sensible and organised friend

We all need at least one of these in our lives. I'm lucky and have a few. These are the fabulous friends who storm in, take charge, don't take no for an answer, and basically take control of the situation. They are amazing and just who you need in an emergency and/or traumatic life event.

They organise school-run rotas, meals, medical-appointment rotas and they take you to hospital time and time again.

They do your ironing and if you don't have anything planned for dinner then they bring something over like a full Sunday roast for four.

They check that you have childcare organised. They run your children around from A to B via C and D. They remind you of school events that you need to know about. They're an absolute godsend.

Genuinely there for you at all times friend

She's the one who holds your hand and listens to everything you need to say. She's the shoulder you can cry on and there for you any time you need her. She sends texts to check that you're alright. In her thoughtful way, she'll always sign off with 'no need to reply.' She's thoughtful, kind and a true friend.

Breath of fresh air friend

This is the friend who waltzes in and out every now and then, bringing a change of conversation and generally being a fabulous distraction.

Whilst having some of the 'genuinely there for you' friend attributes, the 'breath of fresh air' friend also has an ability to distract you from cancer, and the chances are they will get you giggling about one thing or another.

Discreetly considerate friend

This is the friend who leaves food packages, flowers, cards and presents on the doorstep, then sends a text to let you know it's there, but that she didn't want to disturb you by knocking on the door. This friend keeps in touch, offers help and checks up on you, but would never presume to pop in and she doesn't want to bombard you with too many texts or visits.

The 'discreetly considerate' friend is kind, thoughtful and gentle. She's very concerned about you but doesn't want to impose on the privacy of your situation. She is wonderful.

I'm not sure what to do but I'm trying hard friend

Bless her. She's out of her comfort zone but she's stepping up and trying to work out how to help and what to do for you.

She flits between being a 'practical, sensible and organised' friend to being a 'genuinely there for you' friend and sometimes a 'discreetly considerate' friend. She doesn't really know where her strengths lie in this type of situation but she's trying everything and actually, that is where her strength lies. She can be anything you need her to be.

A couple of my friends fit into this category. One friend in particular regularly visits and never turns up without a gift. She also sent me a different parcel nearly every day for a week; microwaveable slippers, false eyelashes, scented candles and boiled sweets because she didn't know how to help me. Whilst all the gifts were gorgeous and helped me a lot, it was her constant consideration, thoughtfulness and that she had my daughter over to her house so often that meant so much to me.

Uncomfortable around cancer but I'll try my best friend

You can't fault someone for being uncomfortable around cancer. Cancer is horrible and it's scary for those people who've never had cancer drop into their lives, or the lives of their family and friends. I completely get that. There's an element of fear of the unknown.

It's especially scary for someone who's had cancer in their life and perhaps lost someone to the awful disease. This is true for some of my friends. Some know cancer only too well and want to avoid it whilst some don't know cancer and they're uncomfortable around it. However, they have all made an effort. They may have sent a card or a text. They may have offered help. They may have delivered a meal for the freezer. They don't hang around for too long, but they're there for you as much as they can be.

Old friends

Friends of, say, twenty or thirty years are particularly special. These are the friends who know you so well and with whom there is a special comfortableness. They know what you need without you having to say it and they know just what to say and what to do.

These friends turn up unannounced on your doorstep the day after hearing your news, because they just need to give you a hug. They know exactly what to say when you're feeling vulnerable and will make a special effort to visit you even though they live in another country or at the other end of this country.

Times like this remind you why you have been friends for all those years. They're like family.

CHECKLIST FOR FRIENDS AND FAMILY

How To Give Emotional Support

- Try to be there for her every step of the way. It is a long old slog getting through the treatment so don't let your support subside. Keep it up for the entire journey, including after all the treatment has ended, which is an emotionally tough time.
- Take your cues from her as to how much she wants to see people and talk to people. Don't assume she wants to be left alone, but don't assume she needs company. She will need both at different times.
- Remember her. Send a quick hello text. Perhaps set a calendar alert on your phone to remember to text every few days or so. Getting through tough treatment can be very lonely, knowing that everyone else is just carrying on with their normal lives.
- Keep in touch. Send cards, notes, letters, emails or texts without expecting a reply. If you write 'no need to respond,' it makes it clear that she doesn't have to reply.
- Be flexible and understanding if she cancels a visit at the last minute. This will probably happen at some point.
- Respect her privacy.

- Don't write her off. Treat her much the same as before she got cancer, so if you're arranging a social event, include her in the invitation. Even though she might not come along, she needs to know that she hasn't been forgotten.
- If she is up to seeing a few friends, then take lunch to her house with a couple of friends.
- Take afternoon tea and friends to her. One of the nicest things that one of my friends did for me was to bring homemade scones, clotted cream and jam for us to eat together.
- Offer to go for walks with her. Take her out for lunch or a coffee.
- Listen when she needs to talk.
- Be a shoulder for her to cry on if she needs it.
- Celebrate the milestones with her. If she is up to it, you could organise something special when she finishes chemo, has had her surgery, or finishes radiotherapy. Be prepared for her to cancel at the last minute if she isn't feeling well enough.
- Look out for her children and partner. They need support too.
- If you arrange to visit her, then do. Try not to cancel (unless of course it's impossible). Visits from friends and family are so important and mean so much.
- Going through chemo is totally demoralising when it comes to looks, so if you are any good with makeup you could offer to give her a makeover, do her nails, assist with scarf-tying and generally help her to feel good about her appearance.

CHAPTER 21

TAKING THE HUSBAND FOR GRANTED

"There is no charm equal to tenderness of heart."
Jane Austen

It's taken a while to talk about my husband, partly because he's just there all the time, through thick and thin, riding the ups and downs, holding my hand and rubbing my back. He's always so patient, riding the breast cancer storm beside me, that I suppose most of the time I take him for granted.

I remember telling him that I had cancer as we sat in the car in the station car park. He hadn't come with me to see Mr Breast Consultant on D-Day because I hadn't been expecting bad news. My appointment was an early evening appointment and my mum had come with me, while my dad stayed at home with the children.

We were arriving home in the car at about the time that my husband's train was due in at the station down the road, so we did a quick detour to the station to pick him up. I needed to tell him then and there. I had to do it before we got home to the bedtime chaos of the children, their delight at seeing Daddy and all the commotion that comes at that time of day. I knew I wouldn't be able to get through all that with this awful secret burning inside me and I didn't want to talk about it until the children were safely asleep.

I don't remember much about that evening, or the next few days, but I do remember him holding me up while I crumpled and he's continued to hold me up throughout the past year.

When I was first diagnosed, I felt incredibly alone, as if I was taking a diversion off my life path, embarking out into the lonely wilderness of cancer-land. I now realise that I haven't been alone. He's always been at my side, constantly holding my hand and walking through cancer-land with me.

From the start, my husband has had this wonderful positive attitude. He's always been unfailingly positive about my treatment and the outcome. One set of very close friends told us recently that at the start of my treatment they looked at him and said, "If he's so positive then we don't need to panic." No, none of us have needed to panic because we've had him around us. He's been a true rock for me. He's kept me sane, positive and realistic.

He's brilliant in these types of situations. He is the person you want around during a traumatic event. He is the one you need in an emergency and he's proven this on many occasions during our almost twenty years together. For example, he delivered our daughter on the bathroom floor, all by himself. She decided she was ready to arrive and she wanted to get out quickly. I only had a little tummy ache and one contraction, then I felt her coming and there was no time to get to the hospital. The ambulance didn't arrive in time, so with the help of the emergency services switchboard on speakerphone, my husband delivered our gorgeous daughter into the world. He wasn't fazed. He didn't panic. It was like he was just going about a normal day's work. Looking after me and the children has become his daily work these days.

He took on Project Breast Cancer in his wonderfully pragmatic and sensible way. He has been to every consultant and oncologist appointment, taken notes, asked the right questions and then patiently talked it through with me on the way home.

He took on the job of telling people that I'd been diagnosed because I couldn't do it. He looked after me and held down the fort at home every evening and weekend that I was unable to get out of bed or off the sofa. He stepped out of his comfort zone to make meals, supervise homework, do the washing, keep on top of the home admin and keep everything as normal as possible for the children. He took time off work to look after me at home on my awful post-chemo days.

He's very sensible and realistic. I have worried and fretted about the side effects. *I have a sore throat; is it a virus or is it just dryness? Do I phone the chemo line? Do I go to the doctor?* He just patiently tells me what to do. He drags me out of the house at weekends for a walk—whether or not I want to—because that is the best thing for me.

He hasn't just been my note-taker, my driver, my hand-holder, my medical jargon translator, my nurse and my supporter; he's also lived through the cancer diagnosis and the treatment with me. His life has been turned upside down over the past few months but he has quietly ridden it out. He's kept his own worries private. He hasn't allowed any cracks to show through his armour.

He's been busier at home with me being out of action a lot of the time and he hasn't had much time to switch-off and relax. No time out for himself or time to spend with friends. He's hardly been out of an evening because that's the time of day when I need him the most—to help settle two crazy kids at bedtime—and he loves an evening out. He enjoys a party, a meal, a few drinks. It's such a big part of who he is. He's a sociable being, and he needs to socialise, but he hasn't had much time for that. He's generally been at home with me and I doubt that I've been much company.

In the evenings, I'm often sleeping or moaning, grumpy, emotional, crying, ranting, worrying. I haven't been fun to be around. I've also been bald, red, puffy, bloated, hairless, eyebrow-less, hormonal and menopausal. Not a good combination for a wife.

Don't get me wrong, of course we've had a few tricky moments over the past few months—cancer can be an unwelcome addition to a marriage and it can most definitely put a tremendous strain on things at times, but his strong presence has patiently been there at my side, unfaltering. During this enforced period of slowing down and re-evaluation, I suppose I've come to appreciate him more and remember why I married him.

 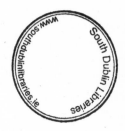

CHECKLIST

Things To Remember About Your Partner's Role In Your Cancer

- Keep the lines of communication open between you. Talk to each other.
- Ask him/her to accompany you to any medical appointments where you need his/her help and support. He/she can take notes, ask questions and then remind you of what was discussed when you later forget.
- If he/she is worried or anxious, he/she can find support from a friend, a support group or one of the online support groups for partners of cancer patients.
- Treatment can affect many aspects of your marriage/partnership. Talk about this together and seek professional advice if you need to.
- The charities listed in the Appendix all have great advice to help spouses and partners.

CHAPTER 22

THE FEAR

"You gain strength, courage, and confidence by every experience in which you really stop and look fear in the face."
Eleanor Roosevelt

Today is a warm, sunny Wednesday in the middle of July. Unfortunately, it's not a quiet Wednesday because it's the school holidays, so the children are at home. As much as I adore my wonderful children, I'm shattered and could really do with a quiet day.

However, thankfully it's not a chemotherapy Wednesday, or a Herceptin Wednesday or a radiotherapy Wednesday. It's my first Wednesday for a very long while without any treatment. Radiotherapy is over! I'll still have Herceptin injections every three weeks for another nine months, and hormone therapy tablets for five to ten years, but the big-ticket treatment is over!

Since finishing chemotherapy and radiotherapy, I've had check-ups with Mr Oncologist and Mr Breast Consultant, at which I was keen to get some sort of cancer sign-off from them both. I already knew that there were no one hundred percent guarantees or miraculous cures, but I really, really wanted some sort of definitive confirmation that:

1. All the cancer had been taken out of me.
2. There were absolutely no little stray cancer cells still swimming around my body that could lead to a spread of the cancer.
3. It would not be coming back to my breast. Ever.

However, it rather unsatisfactorily turns out that doctors cannot give these assurances to quite the extent I was after. To start with, unlike on television and in films, doctors don't give you an 'all-clear' when you finish the big-ticket treatment. There's no marvellous meeting with the oncologist who looks at some test results and exclaims, "You're cured of cancer." No, that doesn't happen.

What usually happens is the oncologist and/or the breast consultant looks at your breast and the surrounding tissue where the tumour originated, and with its continued absence can declare that you don't have any evidence of the disease within you. The original lump has gone. There is no new lump. Ergo there is no cancer.

I didn't have a mammogram at my recent appointments, just the routine of pressing, prodding and pushing of my breasts. No lump was detected thank goodness. The absence of a noticeable lump in one of my breasts at this stage of proceedings was both (a) unsurprising and (b) a relief.

Given a tumour hadn't been found in the first place, had one been found now it would have been a sign that not only had the treatment been terribly unsuccessful, but that there had been a spread or recurrence of some sort of fast-growing aggressive cancer, which my medical team had previously assured me I didn't have.

I would have liked to have a mammogram or MRI just to be on the safe side, but I was told that the mammogram would take place in October, one year after the initial diagnosis. Nevertheless, I had my first assurance: I was told that I had no evidence of disease or NED for short.

In relation to the second assurance that I was after, Mr Oncologist told me that there was no conclusive test that could be done to check that there was positively no cancer left anywhere inside me. I was hoping for some sort of blood test at least.

Based on years of research, clinical trials and the use of treatment on many people, oncologists know how well certain types of cancer respond to certain treatments. Oncologists can state, with a fairly high level of certainty, that if you've been given the appropriate treatment for the type of cancer you have, that it's highly likely that any stray cancer cells will be vaporised (not a word used by Mr Oncologist).

My type of cancer is apparently known to respond well to the treatment I had, which means it's highly likely that had any cancer cells spread further than the lymph nodes, they would've been blasted (again, not a word used by Mr Oncologist). It wasn't the definitive assurance that I was after but it was definitely an assurance of sorts.

As for the third assurance—that the cancer wouldn't come back to my breast—well, that was the subject of a fairly lengthy discussion with Mr Breast Consultant. There are, apparently, some calculations that can be done based on the stage, grade and type of breast cancer, which can provide an indication of the likelihood of the cancer recurring. Given my original lack of lump, Mr Breast Consultant is unable to use the algorithm to calculate my chances of recurrence, so I'm in the dark on that.

However, in addition to working out your chance of recurrence, you're monitored for a period of years after treatment. This involves annual, then less frequent, mammograms and consultant appointments to see whether the cancer comes back in the form of a new lump or regrowth of the original lump.

I won't lie, when Mr Breast Consultant explained this to me, I was a little concerned because if the same situation were to happen to me again then surely there's really very little chance of anything showing up on a mammogram. My original breast cancer didn't show up on the mammogram last year. Nor did it show up on the ultrasound, the MRI scan or on the CT PET scan, but it was there. It was secretly, surreptitiously, mysteriously lurking somewhere in my breast, leaking cancer cells into my lymph nodes.

I have no lymph nodes in my left arm now, so if it comes back and makes its bed in my breast again, how will we find it? I don't have any lymph nodes there to catch the stray cancer cells and raise the red flag of cancer. It's all very well having a mammogram every year for the next however many years, but if it didn't pick it up last time, how do we know it will pick it up if it comes back? This is exactly what I asked Mr Breast Consultant at my recent appointment.

"Well, that's a good question," he replied, as he stroked his chin.

Apparently, it was a question he needed to mull over. He took it to a meeting with his breast consultant companions, which was coincidentally due to take place a few days later. In discussing how to monitor me going forward, there was a divided room: fifty percent thought annual mammograms would be sufficient and fifty percent thought that annual MRIs would be the better option. Neither of those picked up my cancer in the first place so, on hearing this news from Mr Breast Consultant, I didn't really feel reassured.

I was, however, reassured by the fact that when it came to treatment, I'd had the book thrown at me. The chemotherapy, radiotherapy, Herceptin and hormone treatment will all go a long way in preventing a recurrence. Also, if there were to be another lump (or regrowth of the original, invisible lump), the chances are that it wouldn't be a repeat of my unusual situation but would present itself in a more 'normal' way by growing to a noticeable size and being spotted either by me, a mammogram or an MRI.

Whilst friends and family were hugely delighted with the outcome of the recent appointments (i.e. that I'm now officially NED), I won't pretend that I wasn't disappointed by the lack of a categorical, one hundred percent all-clear. In fact, for the first time in this horrific cancer ordeal, I cried as I left the hospital.

I, like many, many other people, have been through hell with the treatment, so I desperately—and quite possibly naïvely—wanted something a little more concrete. Don't get me wrong, I know that I'm hugely, incredibly, enormously lucky and thankful to get a NED result because some people don't ever get to be NED, but it just seems to be more of crossing my fingers and hoping for the best.

Once again, I have that feeling of uncertainty and unease. Bloody cancer. I suppose this is life from now on. The next chapter of my new, post-breast cancer life.

I've let my friends and family rejoice at my NED news. I

haven't told them about my fears. It's as close to the 'all-clear' that they wanted and needed to hear so that they can be rid of the awful cancer in their midst and move on. In fact, many people have asked:

"So, are you all clear now?"

"Have you had the all-clear?"

"Did they catch it all?"

"Has it all gone?"

I completely understand them asking all these questions. They're the questions that I would most likely be asking had it been someone else in my position. People outside cancer-land don't know that there is never an all-clear, but that you can only move forward with a NED. How would they know any different? I certainly didn't.

They think that from now on I will be entering the 'moving on from cancer' phase. In fact, I'm actually entering a phase of 'at least that part is over, now I just have to try to get on with my life knowing that there's a chance of it recurring or spreading'. Recurrence and spread are such ugly words. At the end of the day, it's what those of us who've had primary breast cancer are worried about: will the cancer come back? Will the cancer be caught in time to allow me to grow old with my husband and see my children grow up?

Will it come back as a local or regional recurrence, which is where the primary breast cancer comes back in the breast area and doesn't spread any further than the lymph nodes? If so, will it be caught in time to treat it, blast it, cure it, blitz it?

Or will it come back as secondary breast cancer, which is where the cancer cells have spread from the primary cancer in the breast through the lymphatic or blood system to other parts of the body such as the lungs, liver, brain or bones where they grow into a new tumour? Because if it comes back as secondary breast cancer—which can happen a number of years after the original primary breast cancer diagnosis—then it will be incurable.

You have no control over the possibility of recurrence or spread, just as you have no control over cancer arriving in the first place.

This is Fear and I have Fear constantly perched on my shoulder. Fear has a sneaky way of creeping into my day-to-day life. Despite the positive assurances from Mr Breast Consultant, I still sometimes feel like I'm living on borrowed time and that it's just a matter of time before Breast Cancer comes back again and grabs me in her vice-like grip.

As I hug my daughter, I wonder how many more years of hugs I have left with her. While I'm sitting in the garden with my husband, I wonder how tall the pear tree, a gift that we received when I was diagnosed, will grow while I'm here to see it. As I watch my son play a football match, I wonder whether I'll be watching his matches as he grows. While I'm chatting with friends about the fast pace of life and how time will fly by before the children go off to college or university, I wonder if I'll be here to see that.

With this feeling of living on borrowed time, I feel a sense of vigour about bringing up my children. I want to show them the way, watch them grow, see them become their own people and walk along their own life paths. There's a lot to teach them, to tell them, to help them with, and I don't know how long I have in which to do it. It could be four years or it could be forty.

I've been thinking about how I can take my mind away from Fear, and I have a few ideas:

1. Pretend the whole experience hasn't happened.
2. Hide under the duvet.
3. Binge-watch box set after box set.
4. Run away to a faraway island.
5. Get drunk.
6. All of the above.

As tempting as each of those options sound, they're obviously not realistic, so I'm stuck where I am.

I'm booked in for a mammogram in October, followed by an MRI every other year (it can't hurt to add that into the mix of monitoring) and I'll be seeing Mr Oncologist every now and again. The important thing to remember is that at present, on this particular day, I am NED, which is honestly a huge relief and very, very good news. I will focus on that.

CHECKLIST

What Happens At The End Of Treatment

These points will depend on your hospital/medical team policy and the type of breast cancer/treatment. It's merely to provide an overview of what might happen.

- You'll possibly have a mammogram, ultrasound and/or MRI of the breast where the tumour originated.
- You won't be given an 'all-clear' as such.
- You'll be told whether there is any evidence of cancer from the scan. If there's no cancer to be seen, then you'll be classed as 'No Evidence of Disease' or NED.
- If there's still evidence of cancer, you'll be given more treatment.
- You may continue to see your oncologist and breast consultant at regular intervals for a number of years. This is very much dependent upon your hospital policy.
- Your appointments with the oncologist are to:
  1. Check how you are recovering from the treatment.
  2. Check any long-term effects you might be experiencing from the treatment.
  3. Monitor you for signs of recurrence or secondary

breast cancer, which is where the breast cancer has spread to other parts of the body.

- Your breast consultant appointments are to check the recovery of the surgical site, where you had a lumpectomy or mastectomy and to monitor for recurrence.
- If you have a breast care nurse, you can usually still approach her with any follow-up concerns or questions.

CHAPTER 23

THE LINGERING REMINDERS OF BREAST CANCER

*'In Japan, broken objects are often repaired with gold.
The flaw is seen as a unique piece of the object's history, which
adds to its beauty.'*
Japanese Art Of Kintsugi

We're a week into the summer holidays and the children are both at a friend's house today, which is great because it means that I can have a rest. I'm tired but it's such a nice summer day. I'm trying to fight the need for sleep so I can enjoy the beautiful day here in our improved, neater, tidier and greener garden.

Since D-Day in October last year, I've had my little sidekick, Breast Cancer, right here with me. I have lived with her perched upon my shoulder during every waking moment, unable to shake her off. Despite trying very hard to brush her off, she's never allowed me to forget cancer's enormous impact on my life.

I can't quite remember how it is to feel normal: to feel nothing abnormal or unusual. To just wake up in the morning, get up and get on with what the day holds without having to go through a mental list of how I'm feeling and work out if my body will allow me to do what's planned.

For so long it felt like I had to assess every twinge to work out whether it was:

1. A harmless ailment that would pass without any need for concern.
2. An ailment that needed to be checked out because of my lowered immune system.
3. A non-serious side effect of treatment that I could ignore.
4. A more serious side effect that I should get checked out.

Now that the cancer has been taken out of me and the treatment looks like it has worked, life is about building up my strength and trying to work out how to move on from Breast Cancer. This is easier said than done considering I still have plenty of physical reminders lingering around.

Even though I'm no longer having chemo, I still don't physically feel myself. I can't quite pinpoint exactly why, nor what it is. Yes, the chemo fog lifted a while ago but there's another layer of something hanging over me. It's not the intense awfulness of the chemo fog. It's just something reminding me that I'm not quite the way I used to be.

Sometimes when I go to bed, I feel a general shaking. Nothing visible. It's inside me, like a tiny vibration of all my cells. I wonder whether I'm actually imagining it, that I'm so used to going to bed feeling truly awful that maybe as I lie down to sleep my mind just assumes that I'm feeling awful. It could be an unconscious reaction to switching off at the end of an exhausting day, or maybe the chemo is still in there, coursing through my veins and causing mayhem to everything that it comes across?

Then there's the tiredness. I'm so tired of Breast Cancer and all that it's given me. I'm tired of everything that follows in its wake.

1. I am tired of the treatment.
2. I am tired of all the side effects.
3. I am tired of my never-ending menopausal symptoms.
4. I am tired of worrying and being scared.
5. I am tired of trying to be positive all the time.
6. I am tired of looking different.
7. I am tired of having to rely on friends so much.
8. I am tired of feeling different.
9. I am tired of being looked at with pity.
10. I am tired of missing out on life.
11. I am tired of early nights.
12. I am tired of asking for help.
13. I am tired of feeling helpless.
14. And I am so very tired of being tired.

Most breast cancer websites, books and professionals call it fatigue. I actually don't think that there's a word in the dictionary to describe it. It has impacted every aspect of my life throughout chemo, radiotherapy and still affects me now.

For example, I'm still unable to empty the dishwasher in one go; such a simple action that we take for granted and don't even think about. It takes me three or four attempts to fully empty the dishwasher and put everything away in its place. I unload a little bit, then I have a rest; then I unload some more and have a rest; and so on until I've completed the task and I celebrate by having a lie down on the sofa.

Next on my list of lingering physical reminders of breast cancer is the fact that my body temperature bears no relation to either room temperature or the outside climate.

Hot flushes are a frequent companion these days. A hot flush starts in my upper chest, like a switch has been flicked and suddenly my chest feels very warm. This warmth escalates into a more intense heat and very quickly spreads upwards, to the top of my head, and downwards to my feet, so that my entire body is on fire. Then I sweat. Actual, real beads of proper sweat. There's no regularity to these hot flushes and no consideration for my situation, whether I'm out and about or at home. They just come and engulf me. Layers of clothing are torn off in a rush to ease the intensity of the heat.

As for the night sweats, well, night-time is a constant battle between being drenched in sweat and shivering with cold. I'm exhausted!

Then there are the palpitations. I'm still getting those pesky palpitations that started during chemo. Thankfully, these ones don't have quite the same intensity of those that I had during chemo, but they're still unwelcome. They are also totally uncontrollable. There's no correlation between what I might be doing and getting hit with palpitations. It's not like they come when I'm feeling particularly stressed. They, like the hot flushes, just fling themselves at me with no warning.

Mr Cardiologist has been checking me regularly because I'm now having Herceptin injections and it can, in rare situations, affect the heart. So regular monitoring is normal procedure.

"Well Sara, your heart is perfectly healthy." *Oh yeah, at least something is.* "But you have a floppy valve." *What?* "This really is nothing to worry about. It isn't related to your treatment.

Some people—strangely mostly tall, slim women—are born with it. It's probably a factor in your extra heartbeats. It isn't anything to worry about and it's just coincidental that we've found it now. You don't need to do anything about it for the time being, but it's something that will need to be reviewed every seven years or so, and you may need to do something about it further down the line, when you're much older."

I grinned when he made that comment. I liked the way he talked about a time in the future when I would be an old lady.

Then there is a bit of a weird after-effect. My sense of smell is gradually returning to its normal state. For a time during treatment it was as if the dial for my sense of smell had been turned up to maximum. I could smell something from a mile away, very intensely, and often the smell—whatever it was—would make me physically retch. Anything in the house with a strong scent had to be hidden away in cupboards: candles, air fresheners and essential oils. I had to hold my breath when using hand-sanitiser gel, cleaning products and soap. Worst of all was the smell of the hospital.

On each visit to the hospital the intensity of the smell would stop me in my tracks. The air, a vile mix of cleaning products, medicines and fear, would hit the back of my throat and reach up into my sinuses, causing me to both gag and cringe from the sudden onset of a headache.

The memory of the hospital's smell would follow me around between chemo sessions. If someone asked me about chemo, I could suddenly smell it and would feel my mouth fill with saliva, and I'd have to change the conversation so I didn't start gagging and retching. See, I told you it was a weird one.

You don't even want to look at my nails. All my fingernails

feel as if they've been shut in a drawer and are about to fall off. Some of them are black and brown, but they're holding on so far. This is a side effect of the Taxol chemotherapy, which can be prevented, apparently, by wearing dark nail polish to protect the nail bed from sunlight. I just kept forgetting to do this, so I'm paying the price with my painful, ugly nails.

Underneath and along the top part of my left arm I'm still numb from the surgery. The zapping area across my left breast and armpit is red, dry, sore and itchy, like sunburn. I think I've been lucky with the radiotherapy side effects on my skin because I haven't had many blisters or open, weeping sores like some people experience but just a small area which required some special dressings for a few weeks.

I have constant pins and needles in my right foot and in my fingertips, and thanks to the effects of chemo on my whole body, my skin is still incredibly, painfully dry, cracked and sensitive.

As for my looks, well I'm heavier than pre-chemo. Thank you steroids and carbs. My face is not quite as round as it was during chemo and my ruddy complexion is gradually calming down. I miss my hair A LOT. I still occasionally reach for a hairband to tie back my long hair when I wake up but it's beginning to grow back. I have an almost full head of very short hair but not so much at the front. It looks like an old man's receding hairline but it's long enough for me to be free of the wig and to go out with my fluffy head held high.

I have two five o'clock shadows where my eyebrows should be. The four eyebrow hairs, which stubbornly held on against the odds, are now in the company of many more short, stubbly hairs. It's nice to have my face framed again. Oh, and my eyelashes have returned! They're very short but they're definitely coming through. It's good to no longer have a chemo face: puffy, hairless, bald, red-eyed and ruddy. I'm starting to look a little less ill and maybe a little part of the old me is peeking through.

A couple of weeks ago, on a lovely sunny summer's day, I had some photos taken of me for my website, which has moved from an idea to actually becoming a real thing. I had to be brave for that.

Gina, who is a whizz with a makeup brush, came and did my makeup. She spent a while with me, sponging and brushing and blushing and tinting and toning. For the first time in a very long time, I liked what I saw when I looked in the mirror. It was amazing. A transformation. I didn't look as if I'd just completed six months of harsh chemo and radiotherapy. I had defined eyebrows, cheekbones and colour on my cheeks. I looked generally warmer and brighter.

I put on some nice clothes and in the bright warm sunshine another friend, Caroline, took some photos of me. I felt like a normal person for a little while. We laughed, we chatted, we giggled. I cringed a lot because I hate having my photo taken but I also smiled. These two lovely friends came and made me feel good about myself. I don't think they know how much it meant, or how difficult it was.

It's not just a question of physical reminders lingering. There are also some fairly unpleasant emotional and mental issues that are hanging around. Let's start with chemo brain. I'm fed up with my brain functioning at its reduced rate. I want to be able to remember things without having to rush to write them down before they disappear. I want to remember every single conversation I have with my children, so that they don't have to say, "Mum, I've already told you!"

Not only am I forgetful, but I'm still emotional a lot of the time. I still struggle to get through a day without crying about something. It could be a television programme, radio advertisement, something my children say. I feel ridiculous and I do worry whether I'll always be this much of an emotional wreck.

Then, there is the small matter of anxiety. With the combination of a hormonal imbalance, the menopause and a myriad of chemicals having been pumped into the body, plus the fact that being diagnosed with cancer is an enormous shock to the system, a lot of people suffer from anxiety during and after breast cancer treatment. It turns out that I am no exception.

It isn't just a question of dealing with cancer and Fear, but rather it's a change in the way the brain works. It's a state of mind, a way of life and entirely irrational. When anxiety hits, it's as if all rational thoughts are pushed to one side and replaced by irrational, uncontrollable thoughts and feelings.

Anxiety is different for everyone and it can manifest itself in different ways. My anxiety sometimes manifests itself as thoughts. For example, during a recent visit to a local restaurant, one that I've been to many times over the years, I got myself in a little panic when I went to the toilet. '*If I lock the toilet door then I'll get locked in and I won't be able to breathe and I won't be able to get out and I won't be able to breathe and I won't be able to get out and how will someone know that I am here and how will they get me out and I won't be able to breath.*'

I know it's completely irrational, but as I said, in the world of anxiety, irrational thoughts take over from rational thinking. In addition to anxious thoughts, sometimes my anxiety manifests itself as feelings of unease and panic. It's difficult to pinpoint it exactly, but it's a feeling that all is not right and that something is going to go horribly, terribly wrong but there's nothing I can do to stop it. Again, it's irrational.

When we went to visit the hospital for the pre-chemo appointment, Vicky, one of the chemo nurses, had asked with her head doing that side-tilt that people do when they are saying something to someone with whom they need to be careful, "Would you like to talk to someone about your diagnosis, Sara?"

"Oh, no thanks. I'm doing well and feel fine about the whole thing. Thanks very much."

I honestly was at that point. Yes, I was scared and overwhelmed and petrified to have been diagnosed with breast cancer, but I'd had surgery to remove all known cancer cells from me and I thought that all I had to do was go through a few months of mopping up and preventative treatment to make sure all the little cancer blighters were caught, so that I could jump back into my life where I'd left off. Simple.

So, no, I didn't want to talk to a counsellor and if I did, there was no way that I would tell anyone, not even the nurses.

"Well, that's great," Vicky said. "If you ever change your mind you can ask us because we have a lovely counsellor who sees a number of our ladies here, and we'd recommend her."

During my monthly catch-up phone calls with Shona from HR at work, she'd ask me in her lovely South African accent, "Do you feel like talking about it? Don't forget, we have the on-site counsellor and our chaplain. They'd both be very happy to chat to you about everything."

Always, I said, "Thanks, but no thanks."

However, since finishing chemo and radiotherapy, things have felt, well, a little overwhelming, possibly because I'm only now dealing with the shock of the whole thing. So, I've finally taken Vicky up on her offer and I'm not quite sure if I want people to know this just yet, so shh, don't tell anyone.

Over the past nine months I've allowed myself to rest, recuperate, and rest some more. I've come to realise that it's important to look after me. I have, unlike in my pre-cancer days, listened to my body and gone with what it's told me. I've had to do this so that my body could regenerate and recover from both the cancer and the treatment. I know that I'll need to continue to do this whilst my body gains strength and continues to recuperate. I've made a little promise to myself that, even after I fully recover, I'm going to continue to look after me, to nurture myself.

Despite much soul-searching and deliberation, I'm confident that there was nothing I could have done differently to prevent Breast Cancer making her bed in my body. Having breast cancer has been down to pure bad luck. Plain and simple. It had nothing to do with what I did or didn't eat, what I did or didn't drink, or any other way in which I lived my life. I got breast cancer because. . . I have breasts.

However, I now feel like I have a weak spot and I need to take care of myself so that I can stay as healthy as possible for as long as possible. If I don't look after myself, then I'll be in no state to look after my family. As I read somewhere recently, 'You can't pour from an empty cup.'

All in all, it's taking a little time and some days are harder than others. Sadly, I fully expect that the lingering physical side effects will be here a while longer. Patience has become a steady companion over the past ten months, so I know I can be patient when it comes to waiting for my hair to grow and for the remaining side effects to ease. When I finally reach the other side, perhaps there's a chance that my broken pieces will all fit back together and maybe I can come out a stronger person?

CHECKLIST

Dealing With Anxiety After Treatment

- Stop what you're doing.
- Take a couple of deep breaths.
- Look around and become present in the moment.
- Remind yourself that everything is okay. It doesn't matter where you are just take a second and slowly inhale in and exhale out.
- Repeat as often as required.

CHAPTER 24

THE NEW NORMAL

"To live is the rarest thing in the world. Most people exist, that is all."
Oscar Wilde

The summer holidays are rolling on and today, due to a summer storm brewing, I'm venturing to the cinema with the children. The cinema is always a good choice because I can sit down for a long time, and if absolutely necessary, I can nod off too.

With the harshest part of breast cancer treatment over, I'm trying to enjoy the summer holidays with my children without the cloud of treatment hanging over us. We have a list of fun things to do over the summer; things that have taken a bit of a backseat over recent months:

1. Swimming.
2. The park.
3. Baking.
4. Bike rides.
5. Play dates.
6. Days out.
7. Picnics.

8. Arts and crafts.
9. Sleepovers.

I'm trying very hard to bring some normality back into our day-to-day lives and I'm desperate to find, and step back into, the shoes of 'Normal Me'.

Locating Normal Me isn't just about doing all the things that normal families do in the summer holidays, or going back to work, and moving on from all those side effects that I've mentioned. It's also about getting my head back to the person I was before being diagnosed with breast cancer and back to my way of thinking, working and generally getting through life.

All the way through surgery, chemotherapy and radiotherapy I had a—what I now know to be naïve—expectation that I would return to Normal Me. I expected to finish treatment, get the all-clear, spend a little time recovering from the treatment and then quickly step back into my pre-breast cancer life. I thought that I would just pick up where I left off but now that I'm actually here, it doesn't seem to be going that way.

So much has changed that I don't know how I can get back. Yes, of course I understand that the physical, mental and emotional side effects, plus living with Fear will have an impact on me getting back to normal, but why is it that I'm struggling to return to a pre-cancer way of thinking and living? Maybe it's because there's no returning to Normal Me. Maybe she ceased to exist on October 19th last year, and it's actually a question of finding out who I am now?

So, how has my way of thinking and living changed since my pre-cancer life?

1. First of all, I'm a much slower, calmer person than Normal Me. Gone are the stressful days of rushing around, multitasking, juggling and spinning many plates. Despite it being an enforced slow-down and not one of choice, I actually don't mind that the pause button has been pressed and I quite like this slower pace. Everyone gets where they need to be. Everyone gets fed. The laundry gets done and eventually put into the cupboards. The house isn't as tidy as it once was but it's tidy enough. With a little help from lots of to-do lists, everything that needs to be done gets done. Eventually.

2. Warning: cancer-cliché. Being forced into the slow lane by all the treatment has opened up my mind. I have stopped and thought. I have contemplated, assessed, deliberated, pondered and reflected. I have certainly attempted to put my little world to rights. By opening my mind, I have come to realise (probably rather belatedly in life) that life is bigger than my little bubble. It's bigger than my family and me. It's bigger than my world and this is something that I must remember as I move forward.

3. I know that our regular, busy routine will inevitably resume now that the big-ticket treatment is over. I will once again have to cope with, and balance, my job, my family's needs, our home and everything else that is thrown at me, but I will resume regularity with the understanding that life is not a competition. It's not about striving for perfection or worrying about what other people think. It's about appreciating what I have, not thinking about what I want next.

4. Life is about family and good, true friends. Life is about spending quality time with those I love and who love me. Life is about doing things and being with people who make me happy. Life is about taking it one day at a time. Life is about living.

It turns out that reaching the end of treatment and trying to move on is far more complex than I'd previously imagined and, in many ways, I feel more at sea now than I did during my treatment.

I have entered the no man's land of cancer: the interim period between 'life with cancer' and 'life after cancer,' when the cancer has been taken out and some, perhaps not all, treatment has finished. A time when you want to move forward, but part of you still wants to hold on to cancer treatment as a form of security blanket.

It's a time when you're excited to get on with life, but at the same time you're fearful because you've just spent a significant period of time wondering whether you're going to come out alive at the end of cancer treatment. Your mind wants to move on, but your body can't quite keep up.

I keep coming across a phrase that people talk about when they reach this stage of cancer recovery: 'finding a new normal.' Maybe that's what I'm looking for now?

CHECKLIST

Moving On From Treatment

- Talk to a counsellor, friends, family, your partner and/ or a support group.
- Write a journal, a blog, articles for websites or anything that helps you get the experience out of your head.
- Go on a moving-forward course. A number of hospitals and organisations put these on for women after breast cancer treatment. Have a look at www.tickingoffbreast-cancer.com for suggestions as well as the charities listed in the Appendix.
- Social media has a great cancer community where you can find support and encouragement for moving forward after treatment.
- Regularly check your breasts/surrounding breast tissue.
- If your oncologist/breast consultant doesn't discuss them with you, familiarise yourself with the signs of secondary breast cancer. Yes, it's really scary to think about it, but it's very important to be aware of the signs. The charities in the Appendix have guidance on the signs to watch out for.
- Don't be afraid or embarrassed to see your doctor or

oncologist about anything you're worried about, even if you think it's a small issue.

- Be patient with yourself.
- Look after yourself.
- There are a lot of websites which help people move on from cancer treatment. Take a look at the Appendix at the end of this book for a list of some and also visit www.tickingoffbreastcancer.com for links to these resources.

CHAPTER 25

THE QUIET CONTEMPLATIVE STRENGTH OF HOPE

"Even though everything has changed, I am still more me than I've ever been."
Iain S. Thomas

It's late afternoon on a Friday in the middle of summer. I have a delicious holiday lunch of salad and quiche with a small glass of cold rosé wine in front of me.

I'm sitting in the cool shade of the terrace to our holiday villa in beautiful Mallorca. It's silent apart from the cicada chorus humming throughout the olive groves surrounding us. I can smell that typical holiday aroma of pine mixed with sea air and sun cream. The smell never ceases to take me back thirty years to family holidays in Spain.

The air is a soothing, bone-reaching, soft warmth. It stretches into the shade and warms every part of my being. The umbrella above me is rustling gently as the warm breeze catches it. The sky is a marvellous shade of blue. A blue that we don't have at home; that can only be found in holiday destinations. There are clouds: soft white streams of cloud that blend into the blue of the sky. Through the olive trees I can see the dark indigo-blue of the sea and boats leaving a foamy trail behind them as they pass out of view. The horizon stretches on forever.

Fear, Anxiety and Worry have taken a break today. I don't know where they've gone, but I won't go looking for them. Instead Hope has joined me. She is sitting calmly and quietly on my shoulder. Hope is silent, serene and still. She has been there all along but often she isn't very noticeable. She blends into the background, a wallflower at the party with Breast Cancer, Fear and their sidekicks. She has sat patiently, biding her time for her moment and today is her moment. Maybe the first day of many to come, with Hope on my shoulder calmly telling me that everything is going to be alright.

For the first time in a long time, I feel truly relaxed. My jaw isn't clenched and I'm not gritting my teeth. My chest moves gently up and down with each evenly spaced breath that I take. For once, the heavy weight of Anxiety isn't sitting on my chest. My heart isn't pounding and my skin isn't crawling. My fingers aren't tingling and I can feel every part of my body. I'm not shaking or shivering. I'm just still.

I think that, finally, I've reached the point where I can say that this is the first day of the rest of my life. The first day of being on the other side. The first day of moving forward. The first day of no longer being a breast cancer patient.

As Hope and I sit here, waving Breast Cancer off into the distance, I realise that whilst the whirlwind of a breast cancer diagnosis will leave you breathless, it can also reveal your true strength.

Let's be very clear, cancer is most certainly not a gift of any shape or form. It's cruel, evil and nasty, but I do think it's important that I try to find some positives out of it, or I risk going slightly mad and getting bitterly twisted. I have endured nearly a year of horrible treatment and stress and I'm not even finished with Herceptin or Tamoxifen yet, so if I don't take something from this, I'll feel like I'm letting myself down. I guess it's my way of moving forward.

I took on Breast Cancer, but I'm now ready to move forward and leave her behind. Breast Cancer, as you disappear over the horizon, I have a few parting words I'd like to say to you.

Dear Breast Cancer,

You broke me.

You scared me and you hurt me.

You took my confidence, my peace of mind and my control.

You trampled on my self-esteem, you trod on my composure and you discarded my dignity.

You gave me palpitations; you gave me sickness and the gift of the menopause.

You made me cry. You made me sad and you made me anxious.

You played with my emotions, you knocked me sideways and turned my whole world upside down.

You brought some unwelcome guests into our lives: Fear, Anxiety, Worry and Sadness. But you opened my eyes.

You taught me some life lessons, you grounded and centred me.

You have slowed me down and allowed me to fully take in everything going on around me.

You reminded me how to appreciate.

You renewed my passion for life and my sense of self.

You gave me a realisation of the strength I possess deep inside.

You gave me an understanding of my own mortality and the chance to live life with gratitude for this precious gift.

You gave me a true love for life and for living it well.

I have seen the very best of human nature due to you. Not everyone gets to see that.

Whilst I would have preferred for you to never have come into my life, and I desperately hope to never see you again, I'm also waving goodbye with an appreciation for what I've learnt this past year.

Love, S xx

CHAPTER 26

POSTSCRIPT

"My mission in life is not merely to survive but also to thrive; and to do so with some passion, some compassion, some humour and some style."
Maya Angelo

It's a Wednesday towards the end of March, and nine months since Hope and I waved Breast Cancer off into the distance. I've made a mug of green tea and I'm sitting at the kitchen table with a crisp white sheet of paper and my pencil. It's one of those pencils with a plastic outer case and thin lead running through it and I'm ready to list what I need to do this week.

Other than the sound of the odd car and a few chattering birds, it's blissfully silent here. My husband is at work and the children are at school. There's nobody here at home to disturb me today.

I'm not writing out the list just yet. I'm distracted by looking out at the garden. The garden has that lovely we-are-about-to-enter-spring look about it: green grass, slightly squelchy thanks to the recent rain; trees covered in tiny little pale green buds waiting to explode into lush green leaves. Our laurel hedge, growing amazingly well so that we can barely see through any gaps out onto the pavement. The apple tree, which has sprouted many small branches. They're growing upwards, making it look like some sort of giant spiky-haired creature—not unlike me and my crazy hair regrowth!

The sky is blue with a few large white clouds sometimes allowing the sun to shine through, and other times covering the garden in shade, but nevertheless blanketing everything in a cool spring haze. It's the perfect spring afternoon to be wrapped up warm, inside, with a hot mug of tea.

Today marks a major milestone: I had my final Herceptin injection this morning! Finishing Herceptin is a bit of a double-edged sword. On the one hand, there is no more hiding under what has become my safety net of treatment. Whilst on the other hand, I'm absolutely delighted to be at the end of eighteen months of active treatment and to have the opportunity to move on.

Things have certainly moved on from that day nine months ago when Hope and I waved Breast Cancer off, but I won't pretend that these past nine months have been entirely easy. Sometimes I feel like I'm on one of those long elasticated ropes at fairs that are tied around the waist and then you have to run as far and as fast as you can before the rope suddenly yanks you back to the starting point. I'm really trying to run away, against the resistance of cancer, but it has a hold on me and every now and again it yanks the rope and pulls me backwards.

I've now educated myself more about cancer. We live in a society with an ingrained notion that cancer kills. Look at any television programme, book or film where cancer is a storyline and the chances are that the cancer patient will die before going bald first. For a very long time, since the dawn of modern medicine really, the race has been on to find the 'cure for cancer.' Charities, researchers and scientists are all trying to find the miracle cure. It's been a very long race.

I'm forty-four now and the race started long before I was born. Yet we all know that the 'one-size-fits-all cure' hasn't been found. I mean, look at any set of statistics measuring the cause of death in Western populations and cancer makes it to the top of the table every time. Plus, if a miracle cure were to be found then we'd definitely know about it; it would be bigger than headline news. In fact, there are a lot of different cancers, so it's not a question of finding one cure, but lots of cures.

As a result of living under the cancer-is-a-killer cloud, we as a society don't really talk much about cancer in our regular day-to-day lives. This is especially true of people in my age group (adults under fifty) partly because we all think that it's a disease that affects the older population—which isn't true—and partly because it's so damn scary to talk about dying.

Cancer isn't spoken about unless it rears its ugly head in our lives, at which point we whisper about it and speak of it under our breath, rarely saying the word itself.

Look at me. I couldn't bring myself to write the word on the front of my Project Cancer Notebook for fear of instilling some sort of curse upon myself, and I struggled so much when it came to telling people the news.

When someone passes on the news that somebody has cancer, they tend to say something along the lines of "It's. . . you know. . . they've got. . . *cancer*." The last word is whispered under their breath. Not only is it hard to say the word, but it can be really difficult to be around someone with cancer;

people will say the wrong thing, do the wrong thing or just not show up.

Us regular people, not the researchers, scientists or charities, go about our lives in fear of this horrific killing-beast, ignoring it as much as we can, which naturally means that plenty of us, including me before my run-in with cancer, don't really educate ourselves about it.

The chances are that many of us don't know about a lot of the huge advances being made in the world of cancer medicine. We may not know, for example, that depending upon the type of cancer and how the body reacts to the treatment, it is possible for some types of cancer to be removed from the body and for treatment to be given to help prevent it from coming back.

These people can then live a normal life until they die of something completely different. It's not a guaranteed cure because the cancer *could* come back, but the important thing is that the cancer can be removed and things can be done to reduce the risk of it returning.

Even though it can be difficult to change one's instinctive understanding of something, this is what we need to hold on to. Hold on to the fact that a cancer diagnosis is not always an immediate death sentence. This is what I've been working on for the past eighteen months and I'm making good progress.

Alongside this, I've also looked at various sets of breast cancer statistics. The statistics for someone like me who had primary breast cancer developing incurable secondary breast cancer (also called stage four breast cancer) made uncomfortable reading to be honest.

It made me realise that despite huge advances in getting primary breast cancer patients to a NED result, there is a hell of a lot more research needed to stop breast cancer metastasising (spreading to other parts of the body) and to either cure secondary breast cancer or get all secondary breast cancer patients to a long-term NED result.

Like all things to do with cancer, secondary breast cancer is not a one-size-fits-all cancer with just one type of treatment. There are various treatments and people react differently to them, which means that some people live for a number of years, whilst some sadly die sooner.

Although I don't like what I found out, it was the right thing for me to do at this stage. I realised that a small part of my fear is of the unknown and not knowing the risks. I've made myself aware of the secondary breast cancer signs. I don't want to get too hooked up on these things. I'm keen to move on now, but I thought it would be best to understand the situation and have the knowledge there at the back of my mind.

At the same time, I've realised that I'm going to have to get used to dealing with twinges of pain and not immediately jump to the conclusion that the cancer is back: that a headache isn't brain cancer and a stomach ache is most likely that extra handful of almonds I had this afternoon and not stomach cancer.

Now I'm open to finding out more information about this sort of thing, I feel that I'm arming myself with the ability to set my expectations. I have realised, unfortunately, that Fear will always be with me. It will always be there, sometimes just lingering at the back of my mind and sometimes shouting in my face. Although I will never be free of this fear, I now know that I can learn—with the help of mindfulness, guided meditation, relaxation, talking and writing—how to manage it.

When you feel fear starting to creep up on you, put your hand on your stomach, close your eyes and take a few deep breaths. Look around you. Notice the trees, the sky, what's going on and remind yourself that right here and now you're alright.

"Don't look ahead. Keep present." Those are the wise words of my counsellor.

I've been writing a lot over the past nine months. I wrote this book. I'm writing for my website. I'm writing blogs and articles for charities and other cancer websites. Writing has been a huge therapy for me and it turns out that I absolutely love writing. Who knew, eh?

I've taken what has been a truly horrific experience over which I felt that I had very little, or zero control, and was completely overwhelming, and I've written about every step of the way: what happened, how I felt and what I thought.

I've taken all the chaotic, confused, anxious thoughts that were crowding my brain and put them into some sort of structured order. All this writing has enabled the struggles that I've faced over the past eighteen months to leave my head, allowing me take some sort of control over the whole cancer situation; making it less overwhelming and scary, regaining more control of my life.

By writing about everything I've been able to lift a weight off my chest. There's a saying that by talking about something you can get it off your chest. Well, for anyone who suffers with anxiety, you'll know how it feels to physically have the weight of anxiety pushing on your chest.

For me, the process of writing has most certainly got a lot of that anxiety off my chest. Not only do I find writing therapeutic, but I've also come to enjoy the actual process. I love taking the crazy, chaotic, disorganised, overwhelming, very scary feelings and thoughts going around my head and finding the right words to explain them, in structured, organised sentences and paragraphs. Then ending up with something that other people can read that will hopefully help them.

I'm enjoying social media. I may be in my mid-forties rather than my mid-twenties but I've got (I think) the hang of Twitter, Instagram and Facebook. Although I'd planned to use these platforms to raise the profile of my website and give out the odd word of encouragement to women who are just embarking upon breast cancer treatment, I've taken the social media bull by the horns and immersed myself in it. There is always someone who's been where I am, where I've been, and where I'm going. I've 'met' some truly lovely people from all over the world and together we're trying to navigate our way through cancer and beyond. All those things that I can't say to my friends about cancer, I can say online to people I trust will understand where I'm coming from.

I've been exercising at the gym once a week and out walking every day with our puppy come rain, shine or snow. Yes, that's right, we got a puppy.

During my walks over the past few months I started to think that rather than walking on my own every day, how nice it would be to walk with a little bit of fluffy company. I also thought that, given I was spending more time at home and would continue to do so once I started back at work—because I've decided to reduce my working hours—it might also be nice to have some company at home. My husband and children took no persuading!

In late August, we drove three hours to pick up the most

gorgeous little ball of fluff from a wonderful breeder in Cheshire. This adorable puppy has been the best thing to happen to our family in a very long while.

Buddy the puppy and I have been out walking every day, getting our daily dose of fresh air, exercise and thinking time, building up from short walks to now walking for around three miles a day.

Spring has started to make an appearance over the past few days after what has been a rather harsh winter. Spring, that time of promises: warmer weather, longer days and new starts. Maybe that's why it's such a special time of year? As the grey cloak of winter lifts, we're ready for a change. We feel re-energised and refreshed. We can make plans for the future and we are ready to move on.

Despite my daily Tamoxifen tablet making me feel like an old woman, my energy levels are definitely increasing and I'm actually feeling a lot better. Whilst the lingering side effects from chemo are lessening, the menopause continues to bring joy to me on a daily basis.

I used magnets for a while to try to counter the menopausal symptoms—a simple pair of magnets with one magnet about the size of a ten-pence coin and the other one just slightly bigger. It's called a Ladycare Magnet and you attach it to the front of your knickers for twenty-four hours a day with the aim of balancing the system within the body that regulates the menopausal symptoms.

I know it sounds completely daft but it's honestly a real thing. The trouble with wearing a magnet down your knickers is, well, just that. A magnet in your knickers! It was visible when I wore my gym clothes and it stuck to the shopping trolley in the supermarket. So, when I accidentally dropped it down the toilet, I decided to call it a day.

I'm gradually learning to trust my body again. For a while, I felt completely let down by it. How had it allowed a tumour to grow inside me? All the while keeping itself hidden, and get to the point where the evil little cancer cells had spread to my lymph nodes. I had felt absolutely fine and had no inkling that this was happening.

Since putting my body through such an enormous onslaught of surgery, chemo and radiotherapy, it has regenerated and continues to recover and heal itself. I've learnt that I need to listen to my body: rest when it's tired, soothe it when it's stressed and keep a closer eye on it.

I'm starting back at work in exactly three weeks. Yes, it's been a significantly long time since I was at work but I decided I needed an extended leave of absence to get over treatment and build up my strength. Thankfully, I've had such great support from work that I was able to do this. I know that not everyone is in such a fortunate position with their employer or their business.

For a long time when people asked me about work, it made me panic. Anxiety would jump right up onto my shoulder and I would feel slightly hot under the collar but then, a few weeks ago, my husband and I were chatting about our plans for the year (yes, I know, look at me planning) and it suddenly felt right that I should go back to work. To be honest, there is quite a big part of me that's actually looking forward to it. Back to using my brain, back to interacting with colleagues, back to commuting into London—not every day, mind you— and back to the old nothing-to-do-with-cancer-but-everything-to-do-with-professional me.

So, I guess you could say that one day, without really noticing it, I quietly, gradually, gently slipped into 'life after cancer' and I'm finding my 'new normal.' I'm still me, but a little different. I'm Sara 2.0. I'm definitely still a work in progress, but I'm in a good place.

Although I know I need to do the washing, ironing, food shopping, supervise homework, make dinner, clean and tidy the house, take the dog for a walk, collect the dry cleaning, go to the Post Office, plan an Easter egg hunt, defrost and clean the freezer and get on with all the other wonderful normal jobs at home, I also need to, in no particular order:

- Hug my children and tell them I love them.
- Tell my husband how much I appreciate him.
- Visit my parents.
- Phone my sister.
- Check-in with my friends.
- Live my life, enjoy my life and love my life.

CHAPTER 27

CANCER AS MY TEACHER: LESSONS LEARNED DURING BREAST CANCER

"We all have an unsuspected reserve of strength inside that emerges when life puts us to the test."
Isabel Allende

If there's one thing that has come out of the past eighteen months, it's that I've have learnt a lot about me, about cancer, about people, about life. In no particular order, I would love to share these lessons with you.

I have learnt that:

1. Patience is an art form and it can be learned.
2. We should be grateful for everything and should not take anything for granted.
3. Happiness is precious, so when it visits, savour it.
4. We all possess an inner strength of which we were previously unaware. We are not especially brave, or inspiring, or special, we just dig deep and draw out this special reserve of strength that is sitting in us, waiting for the time when we really need it.
5. We all want a purpose in life and we want to know what

that purpose is. Cancer merely reiterates our quest for this purpose.

6. We should appreciate the here and now, and not be constantly thinking of the next thing. Slow down and enjoy life.

7. You should not allow negative feelings to build up inside you.

8. Kindness is incredibly important and free.

9. You will lose friends during cancer. Some friends whom you would expect to be there for you won't be.

10. You will make new friends and you will also become closer to some friends whom you may not have known so well before cancer.

11. Life is too short to waste on people who don't really care about you and unimportant things.

12. We all need to be cared about and we need to *know* that we are cared about.

13. There is a whole other level of never-before-experienced tiredness/fatigue/exhaustion that hits during treatment and lingers months after treatment ends.

14. Sleep is a rare commodity, so appreciate it when it comes.

15. It takes a long time to come to terms with a cancer diagnosis.

16. It takes a lot longer to physically recover from cancer treatment than you might expect.

17. You get to a point when you realise that losing hair isn't as bad as you thought it would be.

18. It can be difficult when you don't feel in control.

19. There is always hope.

20. There are different types of breast cancer.

21. Treatment for ER-positive breast cancer can induce the menopause and going through the menopause can be unpleasant.
22. Cancer doesn't end when treatment ends.
23. Chemo brain is really debilitating and it can continue for quite a while after chemo ends.
24. People will say the wrong thing at times and it's usually because they don't know what to say.
25. At least one person will tell you they knew someone who had your type of cancer and died from it.
26. Even with the best intentions in the world, nobody knows what you are going through unless they have experienced it themselves.
27. Most people react brilliantly in a crisis and can be relied on to step up, rally around, help and generally be there for you.
28. You will see the best of human nature as you go through cancer treatment.
29. Cancer is indiscriminate. You can do all the right things—eat healthily, exercise, not smoke, not drink and have a healthy weight and still get cancer.
30. Having a scan is the easy part; the hard part is the lead up to the scan and waiting for the results.
31. It can be hard to maintain dignity during treatment but, to be honest, who cares?
32. It is too easy to take things for granted: family, friends, health and life.
33. You are not alone when you go through cancer treatment.
34. Even the most level-headed people can be mentally and emotionally affected by cancer.

35. There are a lot of people who know exactly how you are feeling every step of the way. They are on Facebook, Instagram, Twitter, online forums and at the local cancer support centre.

36. Family is important.

37. Breast cancer does not always manifest itself as a lump in the breast.

38. You can actually shake with shock; it isn't just something that happens on the TV.

39. Telling bad news about yourself to someone you care about is just awful.

40. There is no going back to normal after cancer; it is more a case of finding a new normal.

41. All cancers are horrible, terrifying and not nice to have.

42. Oncologists are nice and not scary.

43. There is more than one type of chemotherapy drug for breast cancer and each type has its own catalogue of side effects.

44. There is a wealth of information and advice available online for cancer patients.

45. Chemotherapy is harsh and there are times when you feel so awful that you wonder whether you will make it through.

46. When you lose your hair through chemo, you lose all your hair! Every single hair on your body goes.

47. Needles are actually not that bad.

48. You don't get told that you are 'all-clear.'

49. Life can be fulfilling, enjoyable and wonderful at a slow pace; it doesn't have to be fast-paced, rushing from one thing to the next.

50. Walking is great.
51. It doesn't matter if the dishwasher doesn't get emptied, the washing doesn't go on, the ironing doesn't get done or if the house is untidy. Life still goes on and there are more important things to worry about.
52. It's okay to ask for help and to accept help. It is all too easy to go through life trying to cope on our own, juggling, multitasking and getting by.
53. Everyone will expect you to get 'back to normal' fairly soon after the end of treatment.
54. It's sometimes hard living with the knowledge that you just had cancer and that even though at the last check-up there was no sign of it, nobody can tell you that it will never come back.
55. Hope is a precious, fragile thing, which can be dashed in the blink of an eye.
56. Life is not a competition.
57. In life, everything changes. Nothing is permanent.
58. It is incredibly important to take the time to look after yourself. You can't pour from an empty cup, can you?
59. Writing is, quite possibly, the best form of therapy.
60. You may surprise yourself in life.
61. You can achieve things if you put your mind to it.
62. Good friends are really important.
63. Look for the positives in life: gratitude, appreciation, love, purpose and strength.
64. Laughter is a good medicine.
65. Life is a precious gift, so live it well.

APPENDIX

There is SO MUCH information, helpful resources and advice out there. It's just a question of finding the right thing for you.

My website, **www.tickingoffbreastcancer** is a good place to start because I've added links to everything that I have found that could possibly be of help or interest to someone going through breast cancer. Here are details of the main charities and organisations where you can find help and advice during breast cancer treatment:

Breast Cancer Care and Breast Cancer Now: the two major UK breast cancer charities merged in April 2019 to become one charity. They still go by their individual names and have their own websites.

www.breastcancercare.org.uk provides information, support and care to people affected by breast cancer. The website provides advice on everything from diagnosis to after treatment, including how to tell children. The website offers information pages, booklets to download or order, a magazine to subscribe to, blogs by people affected by breast cancer, forums where people can talk to others about all aspects of breast cancer, plus a nurse's helpline.

www.breastcancernow.org focuses on fundraising for research. The website provides advice and information on breast cancer diagnosis and treatment together with comprehensive information on what breast cancer is.

www.cancerresearchuk.org is not all about research but also provides plenty of helpful information and advice for people going through breast cancer. They have a good list of resources and organisations to help breast cancer patients.

www.macmillan.org.uk covers all types of cancer, not just breast cancer. It provides advice for all stages of cancer from diagnosis to life after treatment has ended. There are information pages, booklets to download or order, information about support groups near you and a nurse's helpline. There is also a lot of information for people supporting someone with cancer.

www.nhs.uk is vast. The section on breast cancer provides advice for breast cancer patients, from symptoms to living with breast cancer.

www.breastcancerhaven.org.uk is a charity that has six centres across the UK at which they 'offer advice on practical things like money and work, help combatting stress, exhaustion and nausea, advice on healthy eating and exercise. And above all, there will always be someone to talk to about your deepest fears.'

www.livebetterwith.com is an online shopping site stocking hundreds of products to help get you through each step of your cancer treatment, all recommended by those living with cancer. The site also offers stacks and stacks of practical advice.

www.maggiescentres.org is amazing; their centres are located all around the UK. According to their website, 'At Maggie's you can talk to, and get support from, a range of professional people. Our Centres are staffed by Cancer Support Specialists, Benefits Advisors, Nutritionists, therapists and Psychologists who can support you in whichever way best suits your needs.'

www.pennybrohn.org.uk is a breast cancer charity that focuses on living well with and after breast cancer. Their website says, 'As a national charity, we reach out across the country, offering local support, such as free courses and wellbeing events locally, where you need it. Our Introductory sessions and Living Well courses can help you discover the things that make a big difference to the way you cope with cancer. Things like eating well and managing stress and dealing with the emotional impacts of the disease.'

www.shinecancersupport.org exclusively supports adults in their twenties, thirties and forties who have experienced a cancer diagnosis. They offer regional meet-ups and have information by way of blogs, podcasts and video casts on topics relevant to these age groups.

www.trekstock.com is an organisation aimed at young adults in their twenties and thirties who have been diagnosed with cancer and aims to 'deliver practical and social support programmes tailored to the needs of young adults, to give them a better chance of living well through and beyond cancer'. A fantastic organisation.

Finally, I would highly recommend the book *The Complete Guide to Breast Cancer* by Trisha Greenhalgh and Liz O'Riordan. Professor Trisha Greenhalgh, an academic GP, and Dr Liz O'Riordan, a consultant breast cancer surgeon, are not only doctors, but they have also experienced breast cancer first-hand. This book really is the ultimate breast cancer handbook to help you through and beyond your breast cancer treatment.

ACKNOWLEDGEMENTS

I have plenty of thanks to extend to those involved in the journey of this book, from its first scribbled ideas, all the way to where it's ended up. Thank you to the huge range of people who helped me find the confidence to go ahead with pursuing publication. I originally wrote this account without thinking that it would become a published book, but thanks to Gina, Libby, Jo, Charlotte and Kate for reading the first draft and encouraging me to make a move towards publication (and Libby and Charlotte for doing the first edits).

Thank you, Caroline, for your fabulous support of this little project and for putting me in touch with the wonderful Helen and Abiola, who have been truly amazing. Helen and Abiola are 'Hashtag Press,' a boutique publishing house. They are passionate about books, authors, publishing and all things literary. Thanks to them for their belief in this book and their fabulous support throughout the entire publication process. Thank you to my editors, Tiffany and Rachel, for editing and pushing the writing of a non-writer.

Thank you, Emma and Nicky, for reading the draft manuscript from the point of view of a sister and a friend to someone going through breast cancer. Thank you to my new friends Juliet and Laura who read this account to check it would work as a helpful book for people going through breast cancer treatment. A huge thank you to my amazing Breast Care Nurse, Amber, who read this to check for any medical misunderstandings and mistakes, and for everything she does for all her breast cancer patients. Many thanks to those who've kindly read and supported this book with their endorsements: Victoria Derbyshire, Sian Williams, Jackie Buxton and Liz O'Riordan. All of you, as authors of books about having breast cancer, have been an inspiration to me and many others.

I know that usually the acknowledgement section of a book is where the author thanks everyone who has helped get the book from its original concept out to a tangible published book, but I have a huge list of thanks to make to everyone who helped me through and beyond my treatment.

First, thank you to my husband for all your support and generally just being brilliant (thank you for reading the manuscript and being supportive of this book project even though it's meant the laundry has piled up and things haven't been done around the house —we haven't had cancer treatment to blame this time). Thank you to my two amazing children who keep me grounded, make me laugh and give me plenty of reasons for living. Thank you, Mum and Dad, for everything you always do for us, without you we would be lost. And finally, thank you to all my wonderful family and friends who were, quite frankly, amazing during treatment with their practical help, emotional support and general kindness. You all know who you are, how you helped and how you supported us, so thank you from the bottom of my heart.

And, seeing that I have a place in which to waffle on here, I'd also like to make a fuss about my medical team (my breast consultant, my oncologists, and all the nurses and doctors who looked after me) and also all the medical staff and volunteers who work every day in looking after cancer patients across the country. A huge thank you to Breast Cancer Care and Breast Cancer Now. This newly merged charity works tirelessly in every way possible to help breast cancer patients: funding research, campaigning for access to drugs and specialised health care, supporting those going through treatment, and providing all the information someone might need about every aspect of breast cancer and its treatment. They are a true lifeline to someone going through treatment and I am honoured to be supporting them with this book.

And last (but certainly not least) I'd like to make a shout-out to all the wonderful new friends I've made within the amazing social media cancer community. It's worth repeating what I said in the book about these guys. It's like being in a club (albeit an unenviable one). Support and solidarity are on tap. I can post a comment any time of day or night and someone will reply with sensible, comforting words of support and encouragement. There's always someone who's been where I am, where I've been and where I'm going. I've 'met' some truly lovely people from all over the world and together we're all trying to navigate our way through cancer and beyond. All those things about cancer that I can't say to my friends. . . these are the people to whom I can say what I truly mean when it comes to cancer. Thank guys—you are a lifeline to me, and I've no doubt to countless others.

ABOUT THE AUTHOR

Sara lives in Hertfordshire with her husband of fifteen years, their two children and a dog who likes to eat socks.

In October 2016, Sara was diagnosed with breast cancer at the age of forty-two. Not ever expecting to be diagnosed with breast cancer and having to deal with the impact that cancer can have on an already busy life (one involving a juggling motherhood, working and everything else that a forty-something year old woman has to fit in her life) Sara decided to use her experience to help others who were going through the same thing.

Towards the end of her treatment, Sara set up her website, www.tickingoffbreastcancer.com, and wrote her first book Ticking Off Breast Cancer. With the book and the website, Sara has created something that will support and encourage others throughout their breast cancer treatment and beyond.

Sara works part-time in London as an insurance lawyer but now spends a lot of her time working on her website and collaborating with cancer charities by writing and speaking at events.

NOTES

NOTES

NOTES

NOTES

NOTES

NOTES